SPINAL CORD INJURY

• •

Marcia Hanak, BSN, MA, CRRN, received her BSN from the University of Arizona and her MA from New York University. During her nursing career she has held a variety of positions in acute care, rehabilitation, and community health agencies. She is also the author of *Patient and Family Education: Teaching Programs for Managing Chronic Disease and Disability* (Springer, 1986) and *Rehabilitation Nursing for the Neurological Patient* (Springer, 1992). In addition, she has lectured extensively, edited a nursing manual, written two patient handbooks, a video program, a rehabilitation teaching manual, and numerous articles. Prior to assuming her present position as a rehabilitation consultant, she served as the Clinical Coordinator for Rehabilitation at Mount Sinai Medical Center in New York City, the Patient Education Coordinator at the Rusk Institute of Rehabilitation Medicine, New York Universty Medical Center (New York City), and the Spinal Cord Injury Coordinator, New York University Medical Center.

Anne Scott, BSN, CRRN, received her BSN from Columbia University in New York City. During her career she has had a variety of positions in hospital and community settings. Prior to her current position as a rehabilitation consultant, she worked at Mount Sinai Medical Center in New York City as Clinical Coordinator for Rehabilitation, and as the Spinal Cord Injury Coordinator, New York University Medical Center. She has lectured extensively, written many articles, and participated in national, state, and local activities concerning individuals with spinal cord injuries.

Second Edition

SPINAL CORD INJURY

• •

An Illustrated Guide for Health Care Professionals

Marcia Hanak, BSN, MA, CRRN
Anne Scott, BSN, CRRN

Foreword by
Howard A. Rusk, MD

SPRINGER PUBLISHING COMPANY
New York

Springer Publishing Company, Inc.
536 Broadway
New York, NY 10012-3955

First edition published in 1983

92 93 94 95 96 / 5 4 3 2 1

Library of Congress Cataloging-in-Publication Data

Hanak, Marcia
    Spinal cord injury: an illustrated guide for health professionals
/ Marcia Hanak, Anne Scott. —2nd ed.
        p. cm.
    Includes bibliographical references and index.
    ISBN 0-8261-4172-2
    1. Spinal cord—Wounds and injuries—Nursing.   2. Physically handicapped—
Rehabilitation.   I. Scott, Anne, B.S.N.   II. Title.
    [DNLM: 1. Spinal Cord Injuries—rehabilitation.   WL 400 H241s 1993]
    RD594.3.H35 1993
    617.4'82044—dc20
    DNLM / DLC
    for Library of Congress   93-22159
                                                                             CIP

Printed in the United States of America

We dedicate this book to all of the patients and their families who have touched our lives both personally and professionally

CONTENTS

FOREWORD

(In 1983, when this book was originally published, we had the privilege of having the Foreword written by the late Dr. Howard A. Rusk. Dr. Rusk died in 1989. In honor of his memory we have reprinted his Foreword in this second edition.)

Rehabilitation medicine has grown into an important medical specialty. This is due to the growing need for rehabilitation centers that can provide the skills of physiatrists, urologists, nurse specialists, physical and occupational therapists, social workers, psychologists, and vocational counselors. It is the team approach of these professionals that ultimately makes the rehabilitation of a person successful. However, there will never be enough of these centers to provide for those who need them due to the high cost of equipment, staff, and service. Because of this, it is necessary to merge the philosophy of rehabilitation with existing medical programs.

In their book, *Spinal Cord Injury: An Illustrated Guide for Health Care Professionals*, Marcia Hanak and Anne Scott have made a significant contribution to the field of SCI Management, a major form of rehabilitation medicine. They provide information that is applicable to health care providers in all different types of settings. In addition to physiological and management guidelines, they give the reader guidance on how to provide the optimum therapeutic environment that will enable each disabled individual to reach his fullest potential.

I have always remembered the following analogy. It describes the essence of rehabilitation and symbolizes the rewards for both health care professionals and disabled individuals:

Great ceramics are not made by putting clay in the sun; they come only from the white heat of the kiln. In the firing process, some pieces are broken, but those that survive the heat are transformed from the clay into porcelain and are objects of art, and so it is with people. Those who, through medical skill, opportunity, work and courage, survive their illness or overcome their handicap and take their places back in the world have a depth of spirit that you and I can hardly measure. They haven't wasted their pain.

Howard A. Rusk, M.D.
Founder of the
Institute of Rehabilitation Medicine
New York University Medical Center

PREFACE

Spinal cord injury (SCI) is a catastrophic event with far-reaching consequences for the victim, his family and friends, and for society as a whole. Studies conducted by the National Spinal Cord Injury Statistical Center show that approximately 61 percent of these injuries are sustained by young people between the ages of 16 and 30. Males comprise 82 percent of the spinal cord injured group. The estimated population of all persons living in the United States with spinal cord dysfunction is greater than 200,000. The lifetime care expenses for many of them will exceed $550,000.

What can never be measured is the emotional cost. Within a moment, a person who had been active, independent, and in charge of his life becomes immobilized, without control of bodily functions, and is dependent on others to meet basic needs. He will need the support of a well-coordinated team of physicians, nurses, therapists, a nutritionist, a psychologist, a social worker, and a vocational counselor. The team's expertise, concern, and respect for his individuality can help him gain the skills and tap the emotional resources he will need to survive in a society that in many ways may deny his existence through attitudinal and physical barriers.

The purpose of this book is to provide a general informational overview that will assist health care professionals in maximizing their effectiveness within the acute care, rehabilitation, and community settings. While some of the information pertains only to traumatic SCI, most of it also is applicable for any person with spinal cord dysfunction resulting from a tumor, an infectious process, a vascular lesion, or a congenital defect.

There are many different opinions among professionals as to what constitutes optimal care. While we have chosen to present information and recommendations in a direct format, our intent is not to suggest that this is the only correct approach to spinal cord management. For any medical and rehabilitation plan to be truly successful, it must be individualized for the person with the spinal cord dysfunction. To provide this individualized approach, we must be able to recognize and respond to the multitude of psychological, social, and cultural components that have influenced each person's development and will continue to influence future adjustment. To achieve and maintain this perspective, we also must be aware of our own responses and how they affect our interactions with patients and their families.

For most people, the process of adjustment following spinal cord impairment is a long and painful one. Of inestimable value are the health care professionals who can integrate their knowledge with the need and goals of each of these individuals to assist their actualizing their fullest potential.

To simplify the format the masculine pronoun has been used throughout the text, since the majority of persons with spinal cord injury is male. Except in specific urological and sexual references, all of the information applies to females as well as males.

1

NERVOUS SYSTEM
ANATOMY AND PHYSIOLOGY

CENTRAL AND PERIPHERAL
NERVOUS SYSTEM

The central nervous system (CNS) consists of the brain and spinal cord. Associated structures include the surrounding membranes, blood vessels, cerebrospinal fluid, and the bones of the skull and vertebral column. The cranial and spinal nerves comprise the peripheral nervous system (PNS).

Associated Structures

Bony Structures. The skull protects and supports the brain. It is divided into three regions: the anterior fossa, containing the frontal lobes; the medial fossa, containing the temporal, parietal, and occipital lobes; and the posterior fossa containing the brainstem, cerebellum, and the foramen magnum (the point where the brainstem structure changes and becomes the spinal cord). The atlas, a vertebral bone, supports the skull and connects it with the vertebral column.

The spinal or vertebral column provides support for the body and protection for the spinal cord. It consists of seven cervical, 12 thoracic, and five lumbar vertebrae; plus the sacrum, which is composed of five fused sacral vertebrae, and the coccyx, which consists of four fused coccygeal vertebrae.

The characteristic vertebra (see Figure 1.1) has a body, two laminae, and two pedicles; plus four articular, two transverse, and one spinous process. The spinal cord passes through a central opening called the vertebral foramen, and the spinal nerves exit from the cord through bilateral intervertebral foramina. In be-

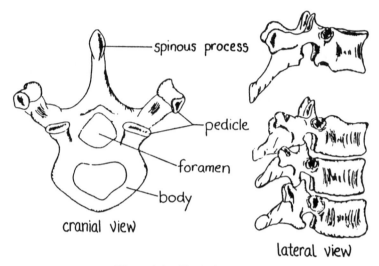

Figure 1.1   Thoracic vertebrae.

tween each vertebra is a fibrocartilaginous disk that acts as a shock absorber. Muscles and ligaments attached to the vertebrae help give the spinal column stability and flexibility.

Meninges and Vascular System. The meninges (dura mater, arachnoid, pia mater) are the membranes between the skull and brain and the vertebral column and spinal cord. They provide support and protection for the central nervous system (CNS) structures.

Oxygenated blood is carried to the brain by the two internal carotid arteries and the two vertebral arteries. The main branches of the internal carotid are the anterior, medial, and posterior, supplying the cerebral lobes. The basilar and vertebral arteries supply the brainstem and cerebellum. The veins from these areas drain into the superior and inferior longitudinal and lateral sinuses, which then drain into the internal jugular vein.

The arterial blood supply to the spinal cord is carried by the anterior and two posterior arteries, which arise from the vertebral arteries at the foramen magnum. These vessels receive an additional blood supply at each cord segment from the lateral spinal arteries. Intradural veins follow the arterial pattern. Extradural veins form a complex network with multiple communications to abdominal, thoracic, and neck veins.

Cerebrospinal Fluid (CSF). The CSF is a clear, odorless fluid formed by filtration of blood plasma in the ventricles of the brain. From the ventricles it flows into the subarachnoid space between the pia mater and arachnoid and circulates over the brain and spinal cord, acting as a protective shock absorber for these structures.

The Neuron

The basic functional and anatomical unit of the nervous system is the nerve cell (neuron). It consists of a dendrite, short branching fibers which conduct impulses to the cell; the cell body, which contains the nucleus; and the axon, which conducts impulses from the cell body. Afferent neurons carry sensory impulses to the CNS; efferent neurons carry motor impulses from the CNS to muscles and glands; and internuncial neurons carry impulses between the afferents and efferents.

The gray matter of the cerebral cortex and the central part of the spinal cord are composed of nerve-cell bodies. Ganglia are groups of nerve-cell bodies located outside these structures. The white matter of the brain and cord is composed of axons, which are protected by a fatty covering called myelin. Bundles of axons have the same origin, termination, and function are called fiber tracts or conducting pathways.

The Brain

There are three main divisions of the brain: the cerebrum, the brainstem, and the cerebellum. The cerebrum, the largest division, consists of two hemispheres covered by the cerebral cortex and joined together by the corpus callosum. Each hemisphere is divided by fissures into four major lobes: the frontal lobe is concerned with personality, behavior, higher intellectual functions, and motor activities; the parietal lobe is associated with sensory interpretation; the temporal lobe contains the auditory center and receptors for taste and smell; and the occipital lobe is associated with visual perception. Other components of the cerebrum include the speech centers located in each lobe, association areas located in each lobe and involved with comprehension, and the basal ganglia located at the base of each hemisphere and involved with regulation of body movements.

The second major division of the brain, the brainstem, consists of four areas: the diencephalon (thalamus and hypothalamus), midbrain, pons, and medulla oblongata. The thalamus monitors sensory stimuli and controls some primitive emotional responses; the hypothalamus has a regulatory influence on some of the autonomic nervous system functions such as body temperature, metabolism, and water balance. The midbrain conducts impulses between the cerebrum and other parts of the brain. The pons connects different parts of the brain and the rest of the nervous system. The medulla oblongata joins the brain and spinal cord, and most of the motor fibers from the cerebral cortex cross over here. The medulla also contains the cardiac center, which slows heart rate; the respiratory center, which controls respiratory muscles; and the vasomotor center, which affects blood pressure. The midbrain, pons, and medulla also contain cranial nerve nuclei. The cerebellum assists in coordination of muscles for movement and balance.

Cranial Nerves

The 12 pairs of cranial nerves comprise the cranial division of the peripheral nervous system into the following:

1. Olfactory
2. Optic
3. Oculomotor
4. Trochlear
5. Trigeminal
6. Abducens
7. Facial
8. Acoustic
9. Glossopharyngeal
10. Vagus
11. Accessory
12. Hypoglossal

They are involved with voluntary and autonomic functions in the head and with the special senses of vision, hearing, smell, and taste.

Spinal Cord

The spinal cord (see Figures 1.2 and 1.3 extends from the medulla oblongata just above the foramen magnum to the upper border of the second lumbar vertebra. A central canal containing cerebrospinal fluid runs through the cord to the lower end (conus medularis).

The central portion or gray matter of the cord contains ventral, lateral, and dorsal enlargements called the anterior, lateral, and posterior horns. The anterior horns contain lower motor neurons whose axons terminate in skeletal muscles. The lateral horns in the thoracic region contain cells that give rise to sympathetic fibers of the autonomic nervous system. The posterior horns contain sensory fibers.

Spinal Nerves. The cord acts as a conduction center between the spinal nerves of the peripheral nervous system and the brain. There are 31 pairs of these nerves divided into anterior and posterior roots: eight cervical, twelve thoracic, five lumbar, five sacral, and one coccygeal. While the upper cervical nerves have an almost horizontal course as they leave the intervertebral foramina, the course of the other spinal nerves becomes increasingly oblique, running almost vertical in the lumbar area and resembling a horse's tail (cauda equina).

The anterior roots conduct efferent (motor) impulses to the skeletal muscles and through preganglionic sympathetic fibers of the autonomic nervous system. The posterior roots conduct all afferent (sensory) impulses to the cord where they are transmitted to the brain via the ascending tracts.

By multiple subdivisions of these anterior and posterior roots, nerves are distributed throughout the body. An intricate network of nerves is called a plexus. The cervical plexus consists of the first four cervical nerves and supplies the neck region. The phrenic nerve, which innervates the diaphragm, is an important branch of this plexus. The brachial plexus is formed from the fifth, sixth, seventh, and eighth cervical and first thoracic spinal nerves. It supplies the upper extremities. The radial, medial, and ulnar nerves are important branches of this plexus, providing innervation of the shoulder, arm, forearm, wrist, and hand. The lumbar-sacral plexus is formed from the twelfth thoracic, the lumbar, and the sacral nerves. It supplies the pelvic and hip region

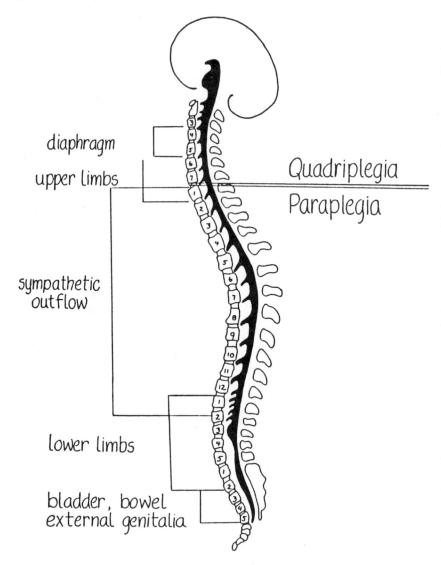

diaphragm

upper limbs

Quadriplegia

Paraplegia

sympathetic
outflow

lower limbs

bladder, bowel
external genitalia

Figure 1.2   Structure and function of the spinal cord.

and the lower extremities. The obturator, femoral, and sciatic
nerves are its important branches. The thoracic nerves do not
form a plexus, but pass out the intercostal spaces between the ribs.
They supply the thoracic and upper abdominal skin and
musculature.

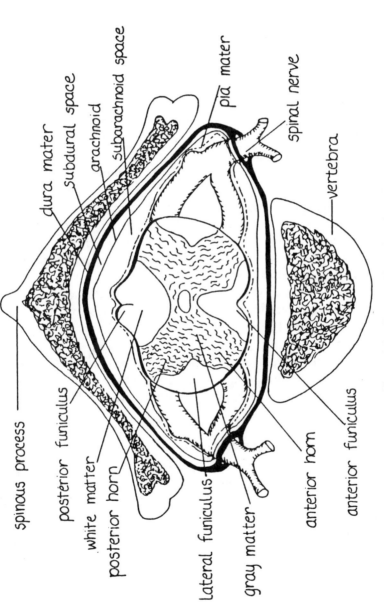

spinous process

posterior funiculus

white matter

posterior horn

lateral funiculus

gray matter

anterior horn

anterior funiculus

dura mater

subdural space

arachnoid

subarachnoid space

pia mater

spinal nerve

vertebra

Figure 1.3   Cross-section of the spinal cord.

Ascending Tracts. Ascending neuron fibers, located in the posterior horns and white matter of the cord, give rise to the spinothalamic, spinocerebellar, and posterior tracts. The lateral spinothalamic tracts convey sensations of pain and temperature from the spinal cord to the thalamus. The ventral spinothalamic tract carries crude touch and pressure messages to the thalamus. The posterior tracts conduct sensations of position, vibration, two-point discrimination, deep pressure, and fine touch to the cerebrum. The dorsal and ventral spinocerebellar tracts carry proprioceptive impulses to the cerebellum.

Descending Tracts. The corticospinal (pyramidal) tracts arise from the motor cortex of the brain and terminate in the spinal cord. The lateral corticospinal tracts consist of upper motor neuron (UMN) fibers associated with extremity movements. UMN fibers involved with neck and trunk movements are in the ventral corticospinal tract. The vestibulospinal (extrapyramidal) tracts extend from the vestibular area of the brainstem to the cord and help maintain upright posture. The reticulospinal tracts also descend from the brainstem and connect with sympathetic ganglia to provide autonomic innervation.

Spinal Cord Reflexes. A reflex arc is the pathway an impulse travels from a receptor (sensory) organ to an effector (muscles or gland) organ (see Figure 1.4). The resulting action is called a *reflex*. There are several types of reflexes associated with the spinal cord: proprioceptive, which facilitate positional awareness; flexor or withdrawal, which follow a painful stimulus; and autonomic, which help control the visceral functions of the body.

AUTONOMIC NERVOUS SYSTEM

The autonomic nervous system (ANS) is composed of a sympathetic and a parasympathetic division (see Figure 1.5). These two divisions differ structurally, physiologically, and pharmacologically.

Anatomy

Sympathetic Division. The fibers of the sympathetic division originate in cell bodies in the gray matter of the cord (preganglionic

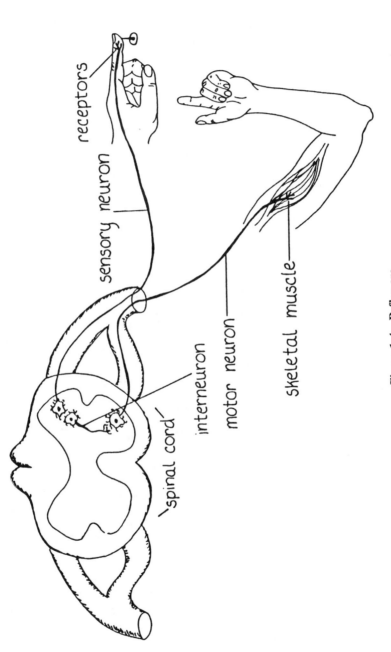

receptors

sensory neuron

spinal cord

interneuron

motor neuron

skeletal muscle

Figure 1.4 Reflex arc.

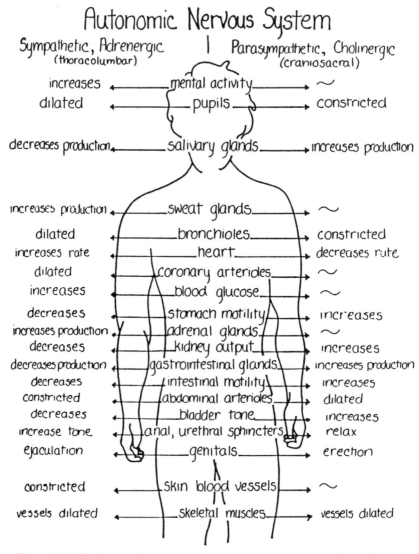

Autonomic Nervous System

Sympathetic, Adrenergic (thoracolumbar)		Parasympathetic, Cholinergic (craniosacral)
increases	mental activity	~
dilated	pupils	constricted
decreases production	salivary glands	increases production
increases production	sweat glands	~
dilated	bronchioles	constricted
increases rate	heart	decreases rate
dilated	coronary arterioles	~
increases	blood glucose	~
decreases	stomach motility	increases
increases production	adrenal glands	~
decreases	kidney output	increases
decreases production	gastrointestinal glands	increases production
decreases	intestinal motility	increases
constricted	abdominal arterioles	dilated
decreases	bladder tone	increases
increase tone	anal, urethral sphincters	relax
ejaculation	genitals	erection
constricted	skin blood vessels	~
vessels dilated	skeletal muscles	vessels dilated

Figure 1.5 Physiological responses resulting from autonomic stimulation.

neurons). They leave the cord through the anterior roots of the spinal nerves. After passing through small nerves called white rami they synapse with neurons in the sympathetic chain (post-ganglionic neurons). These neurons secrete the hormone norepinephrine or noradrenaline. Their action is therefore termed adrenergic (adrenalin producing). Fibers from the postganglionic neurons may pass into the visceral sympathetic nerves that innervate the internal organs or they may return through the gray rami to the spinal nerves. With these nerves they supply the blood vessels and sweat glands throughout the body. To provide sympathetic innervation above the thoracolumbar chain, fibers extend upward from the thoracic region into the neck and to the structures of the head. The lower abdomen and legs are supplied by fibers extending downward from the chain.

Visceral sensory fibers pass with the sympathetic fibers through the sympathetic nerves where they travel into the spinal nerves. From there they enter the posterior horns of the cord gray matter and either cause the autonomic cord reflexes discussed previously or they transmit sensory impulses to the brain via the ascending tracts.

Parasympathetic Division. Fibers from this division originate mainly in the tenth cranial (vagus) nerve. A few also originate in the third, fifth, and seventh cranial nerves and in the sacral segments of the spinal cord. The vagus nerve supplies parasympathetic fibers to the heart, lungs, and most of the organs of the abdomen. The other cranial nerves supply the head, and the sacral fibers supply the urinary bladder and distal parts of the colon.

The cell bodies of the preganglionic fibers are in the brainstem or sacral cord. The fibers themselves pass all the way to the wall of the organ to be stimulated. There they synapse with postganglionic neurons, which secrete a hormone called acetylcholine. For this reason their action is said to be cholinergic. The fibers originating from these neurons travel only a few millimeters before reaching their destination.

Physiology

Figure 1.5 outlines the main functions of each division of the autonomic nervous system. The end result of their apparent antagonistic actions is usually a balanced harmony. This harmony is disrupted during times of physical and emotional stress when the sympathetic division assumes a dominant role. The adrenal release of epinephrine further augments this systemic response. During periods of rest the parasympathetic division has a more dominant role, particularly in digestive and elimination processes.

In addition to structural and physiological differences, the two autonomic divisions have differing pharmacologic effects. Sympathomimetic (adrenergic) drugs prepare the body for physiological stresses by acting on the organs in the same manner as the sympathetic nerves. Parasympathomimetic (cholinergic) drugs mimic the actions of the parasympathetic nerves.

Anticholinergic drugs, by negating the influence of the parasympathetic nerves, have some of the same effects as adrenergic drugs. Adrenergic blockers, by negating the sympathetic nerve response, have some of the same effects as the cholinergic drugs.

Despite the fact that each drug generally is prescribed for a specific use, it usually will affect many other organs as well. By determining whether the pharmacological action is adrenergic or cholinergic, one can predict the other side effects that might be expected. For example, a decongestant has a vasoconstrictor, mucosuppressant action. Figure 1.5 shows that this is an adrenergic action. Therefore, in addition to its primary decongestant effect, it will have other effects such as increasing heart rate and blood pressure and decreasing bowel and bladder tone.

2

NEUROLOGICAL TRAUMA

ETIOLOGY

Trauma to the head, neck, shoulders, or back resulting from a fall, a motor vehicle or sports accident, or a penetrating wound may cause injury to the vertebral column, to the spinal cord, or to both.

Vertebral Injuries

The degree and type of force that is exerted on the spine at the time of the accident will be determining factors in whether a vertebral injury occurs (see Figures 2.1 through 2.4). Damage to the ligaments, which help to stabilize the vertebral column, will cause further instability. Sudden hyperflexion and rotation, as seen in many motor vehicle accidents, frequently result in a fracture dislocation with C_{5-6} and T_{12}-L_1 being the most common sites. This is an unstable fracture due to posterior longitudinal ligament damage, and it usually causes the greatest degree of cord damage. High-impact longitudinal trauma, as seen after a long-distance fall, often will result in a compression fracture. This is a more stable fracture as the posterior ligament and posterior bony elements remain intact. The most common sites are also C_{5-6} and T_{12}-L_1. Neurological damage usually is less extensive with this type of fracture. A hyperextension injury from a fall or motor vehicle accident is seen most often in the older person with degenerative changes in the spine. C_{4-5} is the most common site. Skeletal damage is seen in the anterior ligament rather than in the vertebral column. If neurological damage occurs it usually involves the center of the cord.

Neuropathology and Related Research

As indicated previously, varying degrees of spinal cord damage usually accompany vertebral fractures and dislocations; however,

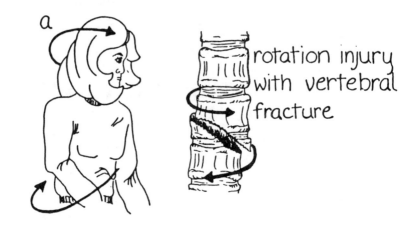

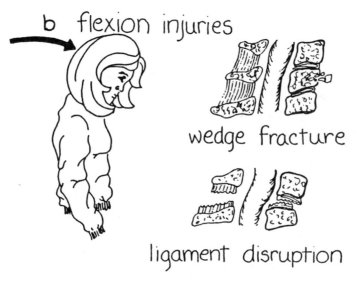

Figure 2.1   Injuries causing damage to the spinal cord.

not all spinal cord injuries are associated with vertebral injuries. The cord may be lacerated by a bullet or knife wound or sustain a concussion or contusion following a high-impact accident.

The spinal cord is rarely physically transected by any of these injuries. The damage results from an autodestruction process that begins at the time of the initial insult. At the time, petechial hemorrhages occur in the gray matter. Within 1 to 2 hours, extravasa-

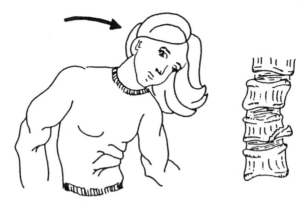

Figure 2.2   Lateral flexion injuy resulting in wedge fracture of the vertebra.

tion of fluid, red blood cells, and lymphocytes extend through the gray matter. The hemorrhages, edema, and metabolic products acting together result in ischemia and necrosis of the spinal neurons. In response to the trauma the body increases the production of norepinephrine and endorphins. These, in turn, cause vascular changes which result in further hypoxia and necrosis. Within 4 hours after injury 40 percent of the gray matter and adjacent white matter at the injury site may be necrosed. Within 24 hours the continuation of the destructive process results in extensive ne-

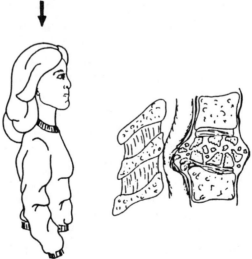

Figure 2.3   Vertical compression injury resulting in burst vertebral body.

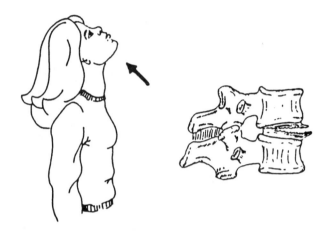

Figure 2.4   Hyperextension injury disrupting the intervertebral disc.

crotic changes. Edema secondary to the inflammatory process compresses the cord and further increases the ischemic damage. While there is usually a stabilization of the destructive processes within 48 hours, progressive edema can extend the damage up to 72 hours.

Many research projects are being conducted currently in an attempt to isolate these destructive factors and develop treatments to counteract their effects. The following experimental methods are being used at various medical centers in the United States: Alpha methytyrosine (AMT), reserprine, or levodopa to counteract the effects of norepinephrine; naloxone or thyrotropin releasing hormone (TRH) to counteract the effects of the catecholamines and endorphins, calcium channel blockers combined with dextrate to counteract the loss of blood to the cord, and 21 aminosteroids to counteract the production of free radicals.

In 1990, the National Institute of Health released the results of a several year multicenter study of the use of methylprednisolone. When given within 8 hours of injury, high intravenous doses of this drug (given over a period of 24 hrs.) can reduce the motor and sensory losses associated with SCI. It is thought to act by stabilizing nerve cell membranes and protecting them from further injury after the initial trauma.

Other modalities under investigation include GM-1 ganglioside to promote outgowth of neurites, peripheral nerve grafts to enhance the regrowth environment, omentum transfer to enhance circulation and facilitate nerve cell growth, administration of nerve growth factor and thyroid hormones to increase anabolic actions, fetal tissue transplants to replace neurons, and electrical stimulation to enhance neuron growth. There is no conclusive evidence in support of any of these modalities at the present time.

TYPES OF SPINAL CORD INJURY

Motor Neuron and Disability Classification

Injuries may be classified as upper motor neuron (UMN) or lower motor neuron (LMN). An UMN lesion occurs above T12/L1 and disrupts motor axons in the corticospinal tracts resulting in paralysis and increased muscle tone below the level of injury and intact reflexes which are not influenced by supraspinal control. A LMN lesion occurs at or below L1 or in a central or longitudinal cord injury resulting in a flaccid paralysis below the level of injury, disrupting reflex arcs, and absent reflexes. A mixed injury occurs at T12/L1 with manifestations such as flaccid bladder and spastic sphincter or spastic lower extremities and flaccid bladder.

ASIA Impairment Scale

The following scale is used in grading the degree of impairment:

A[5] **Complete**: No motor or sensory function is preserved in the sacral segments S4–S5.

B[5] **Incomplete**: Sensory but not motor function is preserved below the neurological level and extends through the sacral segments S4–S5.

C[5] **Incomplete**: Motor function is preserved below the neurological level, and the majority of key muscles below the neurological level have a muscle grade less than 3.

D[5] **Incomplete**: Motor function is preserved below the neurological level, and the majority of key muscles below the neurological level have a muscle grade greater than or equal to 3.

E[5] **Normal**: Motor and sensory function is normal.

Clinical Syndromes

Incomplete injuries are further categorized according to the area of damage: central, lateral, anterior, or peripheral. A *Central Cord Syndrome* results when there is more cellular destruction in the center of the cord than in the periphery. There is sensory sacral sparing and greater weakness in the upper extremities, as these nerve tracts are more centrally located than those for the lower extremities. This syndrome is often seen in older people in whom arthritic changes have caused a narrowing of the spinal canal. In such cases, cervical hyperextension without vertebral fracture may precipitate central cord damage.

A *Brown-Sequard Syndrome* results when primarily only one side of the cord is damaged, as in a stabbing or gunshot injury. Below the level of injury there is relatively greater motor loss and loss of proprioception on the ipsilateral side, a loss of pain and temperature sensitivity on the contralateral side.

An *Anterior Spinal Cord Syndrome* results from a flexion injury that damages the anterior spinal artery or the anterior aspect of the cord. There is paralysis and loss of pain, temperature, and touch sensation. Proprioception and position sense are preserved.

A *Cauda Equina Syndrome* involves injury to the lumbo-sacral nerve roots within the neural canal. It results in areflexic bowel and bladder and lower limbs with lesions as in C on the impairment scale.

A *Conus Medullaris Syndrome* involves injury of the sacral cord (conus) and lumbar nerve roots within the neural canal. It usually results in an areflexic bowel and bladder and lower limbs with lesions as in B on the impairment scale. Sacral segments may occasionally show preserved reflexes, e.g., bulbocavernosus and micturition with lesions as in A on the impairment scale.

Additional Classifications

Quadriplegia (tetraplegia) refers to impairment or loss of motor and/or sensory function in the cervical segments of the cord due to neural element damage within the spinal canal. Quadriplegia results in functional impairment in the arms, legs, trunk, and pelvic organs.

Paraplegia refers to impairment or loss of motor and/or sensory function in the thoracic, lumbar, or sacral segments of the cord due to neural element damage within the spinal canal. With paraplegia arm function is spared but, depending on the level of injury, trunk, legs, and pelvic organs may be involved.

Use of the terms quadriparesis and paraparesis is discouraged as the ASIA Impairment Scale provides more precise descriptions of incomplete lesions.

AUTONOMIC MANIFESTATIONS

Since the divisions of the nervous system are structurally and functionally interconnected, damage to one division also will affect the other divisions. This is demonstrated clearly by the autonomic dysfunction that occurs following an SCI. The level and severity of the injury are important factors in determining the extent of this dysfunction.

Spinal Shock

Within 30 to 60 min. following spinal cord trauma autonomic and motor reflexes below the level of injury are suppressed. This areflexic state is called *spinal shock* and may last hours to weeks. The cause is thought to be due in part to the sudden cessation of efferent impulses from the supraspinal centers. The effect of this condition on various bodily functions will be explained in subsequent chapters. Recovery from spinal shock begins with the return of any previously absent reflex activity.

Cardiovascular Effects

The interruption of brainstem communication with the sympathetic neurons leads to systemic vasodilatation and cardiac slowing. Conditions resulting from the vasodilatation include vasomotor shock, postural hypotension, and lower-extremity edema (see Chapter 5).

Thermoregulation

Internal temperature control is an interrelated system between the hypothalamus, the autonomic nervous system, and the cardiovascular system. As discussed previously, one of the effects of autonomic (sympathetic) disruption is vasodilatation. These dilated vessels no longer can assist in internal thermoregulation by responding to heat with increased vasodilatation or to cold with vasoconstriction.

Sweating is another autonomic component of thermoregulation that is disrupted. Instead of helping to cool the body, it occurs as a response to other sensory stimuli such as a distended bladder.

Because of these various changes the person with SCI will assume the temperature of the environment (poikilothermia). Therefore, external temperature extremes must be avoided and high fevers treated with external cooling methods.

Gastrointestinal and Urological Effects

Interruption of sympathetic innervation to the gastrointestinal system leaves the vagal action of hydrochloric acid production unopposed. The spinal cord injured individual is then more susceptible to ulcers and gastrointestinal bleeds.

The sudden interruption of parasympathetic and sympathetic innervation to the bowels and bladder immediately following the injury will result in a flaccid paralysis. As spinal shock resolves, autonomic responses will play an important role in formulating management plans (see Chapters 8 and 9).

Autonomic Hyperreflexia

Autonomic hyperreflexia (dysreflexia) is a potentially life threatening condition encountered in individuals with spinal cord lesions above T_6 (see Figure 2.5). It is the result of increased autonomic activity caused by a noxious stimulus below the level of injury. This stimulus is most often a distended bladder or bowel. Urinary stones, severe bladder infections, decubitus ulcers, and ingrown toenails are some of the other stimulants that may initiate the autonomic response.

Impulses then travel from the receptor (site of the stimulant) up the spinothalamic and posterior columns until they are blocked at the level of the lesion. Concurrently, local vasoconstrictive responses are activated and the individual experiences a

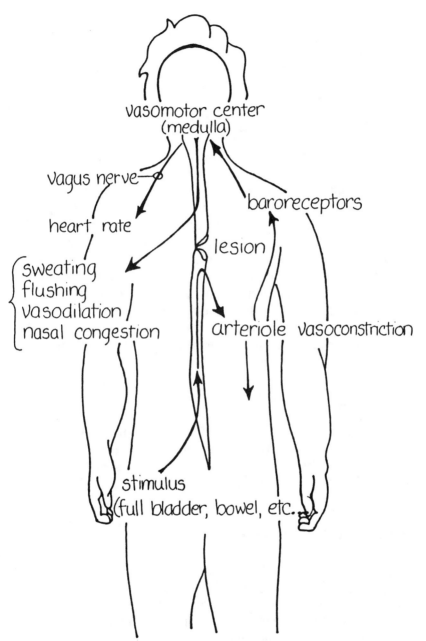

Figure 2.5 Physiologic response during autonomic hyperreflexia.

severe headache as his blood pressure rapidly rises. The hypertension is detected by the baroreceptors in the aortic arch, carotid sinus, and vasomotor center of the medulla. The vasomotor center than sends parasympathetic impulses via the vagus nerve in an attempt to lower the blood pressure. The resulting vasodilatation causes the individual to become flushed, sweat profusely above the lesion level, and develop nasal congestion. The vagus stimulation will cause cardiac slowing.

Because these parasympathetic impulses cannot travel down the cord past the lesion, their effects are only manifested above this level and the sympathetic vasoconstrictive response will continue to elevate the blood pressure. This greatly elevated pressure can result in convulsions and cerebral hemorrhage. Therefore, when any warning symptoms appear, take immediate action to determine the cause and remove the noxious stimulant.

Relieve any distention with caution, to avoid further stimulation. If a bowel disimpaction is necessary, provide lubrication with a local anesthetic jelly. If the noxious stimulant cannot be removed easily, as in the case of cystitis, an anticholinergic medication may be helpful in relaxing the bladder while appropriate treatment is given for the underlying cause.

Horner's Syndrome

Paralysis of the cervical portion of the sympathetic chain will result in pupil constriction and absence of sweating and vasodilatation on the affected side. This condition is called *Horner's Syndrome*. No specific treatment is available.

SENSORY CHANGES AND PAIN

Interruption of the ascending sensory fibers causes an immediate loss of sensation following an SCI. As the phase of spinal shock resolves, various patterns of recovery may become evident in those patients with incomplete lesions, usually beginning the sacral area and moving in an ascending direction.

The pain syndromes of SCI have been classified into four types: mechanical, peripheral, visceral, and central. Mechanical pain usually occurs at the level of injury and most commonly originates from damaged facet joints or nonunion of spinal fracture. It is a dull ache aggravated by movement. This type of pain is managed by analgesics, muscle strengthening activities, positioning modifications, external orthoses, and rest.

Peripheral (segmental) pain arises from peripheral nerve damage. It is a sharp, shooting, radicular pain. It usually follows the segmental distribution of the nerve root of origin. Local measures such as protection from tactile stimulation may provide some relief. However, this type of pain is generally difficult to treat. Medical procedures such as nerve blocks and sympathectomies have been tried with only limited success.

Visceral pain is often precipitated by distension of an abdominal viscus. The pain is transmitted via sympathetic pathways to the high thoracic cord. It is usually felt in the anterior chest, epigastrium, or suprapubic region. Primary preventive measures include well-managed bowel and bladder programs.

Central (deafferentation) pain arises from the spinal cord itself as a result of the major disruption in normal pain transmission pathways and reorganization of neural mechanisms. Segmental pain occurs at the level of injury and phantom pain is perceived below the level of injury in the area of sensory loss. It may be constant or intermittent. It is often aggravated by pressure sores, urinary tract infections, distended bowel and bladder, and prolonged sitting.

In addition to the preventive measures discussed previously, antidepressant and antipsychotic medications have been found to be particularly helpful in SCI pain syndromes. Antispasticity and anticonvulsant medications may also be helpful in alleviating or reducing SCI related pain. For some individuals transcutaneous electrical nerve stimulation (TENS) may provide transient or long term pain relief. Most surgical procedures such as neurectomies and rhizotomies have not been effective in alleviating pain. However, recently a procedure which selectively destroys areas of the dorsal horns (radiofrequency dorsal root entry zone lesion) has shown promise in thoracolumbar injuries with segmental or phantom pain in the legs.

3

EMERGENCY MANAGEMENT

THE ACCIDENT SITE

A quick but complete assessment is imperative at the scene of any accident in order to determine the extent of injury and establish priorities for care, since any life-threatening condition demands immediate attention. The following guidelines review general emergency management procedures with modifications given for the victim with a possible spinal cord injury (SCI). This would involve any individual who has sustained trauma to the face, head, neck, shoulders, or back. Complaints of pain or spasm in any of these areas and loss of sensation and/or mobility are additional warning signs indicating a possible SCI. Any person found unconscious following a traumatic accident should be handled as if he had an SCI and should not be moved without expert help unless there is immediate danger of fire or explosion. Many potential or partial injuries have become permanent disabilities because incorrect handling at the scene of the accident caused further spinal cord trauma.

Cardiorespiratory Resuscitation

Initially, the caregiver at the scene of the accident must assess the victim's respiratory and cardiac status:

1. If he is unresponsive, activate the EMS system, then check for spontaneous respiration. Listen for breath sounds; look for chest movement (rise and fall); feel for air movement from the nose or mouth.
2. If he is having difficulty breathing, keep his head and neck immobile and check for and remove any airway obstruction.
3. If breathing is not restored, perform mouth-to-mouth resuscitation. A modified jaw-thrust maneuver may be utilized,

where the rescuer places his hands on either side of the victim's head to maintain neutral alignment and then uses the index fingers to displace the jaw forward. If this is unsuccessful, *gently* extend the head and neck with a *slight* lifting motion and pull the jaw forward to open the airway. Do not tilt the head back too far, and never let the head fall forward. (With two rescuers the second rescuer ensures that the cervical spine is absolutely stabilized in the neutral position during the jaw-thrust maneuver.) Once the airway is open, pinch the nose and, with a tight seal over the victim's mouth, blow into it four times in succession. Observation of chest movement will indicate lung expansion.

4. While maintaining the head position with one hand, palpate the carotid pulse with the other. If the pulse is absent, commence external cardiac compression. Place the heel of one hand on the lower half of the sternum, two finger widths above the xiphoid; place the other hand on top, and depress the sternum 1.5 to 2 in. for an adult (Do not allow fingers to touch chest.) Between compressions release pressure on the sternum, but do not remove the hands, thus maintaining proper hand placement.

5. For a single rescuer, the ratio of compressions to respirations is 15:2, with a compression rate of 80 to 100 per min. For a two-person rescue, the ratio is five compressions to one ventilation at a rate of 80 to 100 compressions per min.

6. Check pupil reaction and carotid pulse periodically to determine effectiveness of efforts.

7. When cardiac compression is needed, spinal column immobilization may be sacrificed. In an attempt to avoid further cord damage, maintain spinal alignment during any necessary position changes. If you use a board or any other firm surface under the person to facilitate compression, this also should provide some protection of the spinal column during the procedure.

Water Injuries

In water accidents different techniques are needed, depending on the individual circumstances.

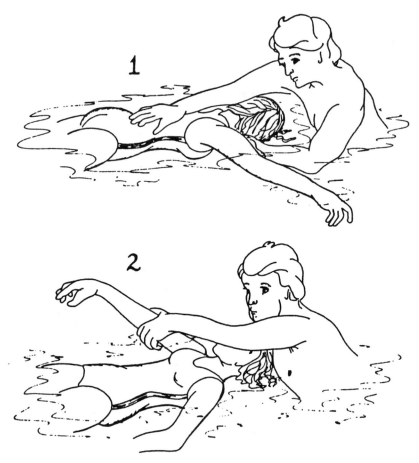

Figure 3.1   Water rescue.

1. Do not remove the victim from the water until a rigid support such as a door or surfboard has been obtained and until there are enough people to assist.
2. If he is floating face down, place one of your hands in the middle of his back and your other hand under his upper arm (see Figure 3.1).
3. Gently rotate him to a face-up position while maintaining his head and body in alignment with his head supported between your forearms.
4. If mouth-to-mouth resuscitation is needed, begin it in this

position using a jaw-thrust maneuver to open the airway without tilting his head. Then float the board under him and use any available material to secure his body in position before lifting him from the water.

5. When no support is available, tow the victim to shallow water with one of your hands supporting the back of his neck and the other hand at his back.

6. Always keep his head and back in alignment and coordinate movements of all rescuers for a smooth lift from the water to a firm surface.

Controlling Blood Loss

The victim may demonstrate symptoms of shock from blood loss (hypotension and tachycardia). To control bleeding, use a sterile compression dressing over the wound site. If this is not sufficient, use digital pressure over the arterial supply to the wound area. For example, if the wound is on the thigh, pressure would be applied to the ipsolateral femoral artery and the leg would be elevated if possible. The use of tourniquets should be reserved as a last resort.

Neurological Assessment

After evaluating and successfully carrying out any of the previously discussed life-support measures, give the injured person a basic neurological evaluation to establish a baseline. Be extremely careful that motor function testing of the extremities does not compromise spinal alignment or exacerbate any other medical complications. Record the levels of sensation and voluntary motion. In addition, outline the level of sensation on the victim to facilitate future assessments. For further explanation of neurological testing and injury levels, see Chapters 4 and 11.

TRANSPORT TO HOSPITAL

The injured person must be prepared properly for transport to a hospital (see Figure 3.2).

1. In either cervical or back injuries, never move the person until adequate help is available and appropriate immobili-

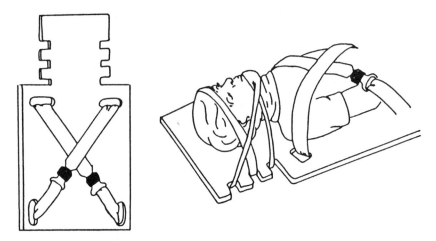

Figure 3.2   Backboard used for emergency stabilization.

zation equipment secured (long, wide board, door, stretcher).

2. Roll him partly on his side, keeping his head and back in straight alignment. Slide the board under him and return him to the supine position.

3. Arrange rolled blankets or clothing on both sides of his head, neck, and trunk for immobilization; further immobilize his neck with a cervical collar if one is available; secure him to the board.

4. Never manipulate or try to straighten any spinal deformity unless it is absolutely necessary to restore an airway. Do not attempt to remove any headgear, such as a helmet, without a physician in attendance.

5. Monitor his respiratory, circulatory, and neurologic status throughout the transport.

6. If the injured person demonstrates signs of vasomotor shock (hypotension and bradycardia), place him, gently, in the Trendelenburg position while maintaining spinal alignment (see Chapter 5).

7. If nausea or vomiting occur, tilt the person (on the board) to the side to prevent aspiration of stomach contents.

IN THE EMERGENCY DEPARTMENT

Once the person with spinal cord injury has been transferred to the hospital, the goals continue to focus on resolving any life-threatening situations that have occurred with or as a result of the injury and on maintaining spinal column stabilization.

Monitor neurological vital signs frequently. If the patient demonstrates symptoms of shock, make a careful diagnosis to determine whether the low blood pressure is due to a massive bleed (hypovolemic shock) or whether it is due to massive vasodilatation secondary to loss of sympathetic tone (vasomotor shock). Unless both situations exist simultaneously, bradycardia rather than tachycardia will accompany the hypotension of vasomotor shock. The patient should be placed on a cardiac monitor, as rate changes and irregularities may indicate the need for further intervention measures.

Overhydration can complicate his condition further by causing pulmonary edema and possibly exacerbating the edema that occurs in the spinal cord in the initial hours following the injury. Therefore, administer intravenous fluids at a carefully monitored rate to maintain the systolic pressure above 100 mg Hg and urinary output of 30 cc per hr. (see Chapter 5).

A primary concern if the person has sustained a cervical injury is the interruption of automatic respiration due to partial or complete loss of intercostal and diaphragm innervation. Carefully assess his respiratory efficiency through the use of blood gases, vital signs, vital capacity, tidal volume, and visual evaluation of type of chest wall motion, quality of breathing, and skin and nailbed color to determine whether oxygenation, intubation, and ventilatory support are needed (see Chapter 6).

In addition to loss of vasomotor tone, there is a complete or nearly complete suppression of all other reflexes, resulting in loss of temperature control, paralytic ileus, and flaccid bladder. This spinal shock is thought to be caused by the sudden cessation of efferent impulses and by inadequate microcirculation to the cord. It may last for days or weeks, depending on the level and severity of the injury.

Insert a nasogastric tube and aspirate gastric contents to prevent abdominal distention from interfering with a diaphragm motion and further compromising respiratory function. Details of nutrition and gastrointestinal management will be discussed in Chapters 7 and 9.

Prevent overdistention of the flaccid bladder by inserting an indwelling catheter or by initiating an intermittent catheterization program. Details of urinary management and other preventive measures will be discussed further in Chapter 8.

A number of metabolic disturbances may occur as a result of the injury or from complications associated with the injury. These include hypernatremia, hypokalemia, and increased endogenous release of steroids. Management of these and other metabolic and electrolyte disturbances will be discussed in Chapters 5, 7, and 9.

4

NEUROLOGICAL MANAGEMENT

For the patient with a spinal cord injury, preventing further neurological damage remains a primary consideration. Until the final stabilization plan has been instituted, move him as little as possible. When transfer from the initial transport board becomes necessary in the hospital, a special lifting device such as a Surglift® can be used. If such a device is unavailable, secure an adequate number of people to lift his body as one unit while maintaining spinal alignment.

DIAGNOSTIC STUDIES

As indicated in Chapter 3, subjective symptoms of SCI may include a combination of the following, depending on the level and severity of the damage: (1) loss of sensation and motor function, (2) pain and muscle spasm at the level of the lesion, (3) loss of bowel and bladder control, and (4) respiratory distress in patients with higher lesions. Many diagnostic studies are needed to determine objectively the type and extent of spinal cord damage.

Neurological Examination

Perform careful neurological assessments at frequent intervals. These assessments should include level of consciousness and pupillary reaction, as a head injury may have occurred along with the SCI. Signs of any increasing or decreasing deficits are crucial prognostic and management indicators.

With a motor examination, identify the highest spinal cord segment associated with diminished motor function and determine whether or not there is any scattered motor function below this level. The major muscle groups associated with each segment are reviewed in Chapter 11. Also record whether the movement is strong or weak when tested against resistance.

As with the motor examination, identify the highest level of impaired sensation and whether there are any areas of intact sensation below this level. Test light touch with cotton, following the dermatomal pattern (Figure 4.1). Test joint position sense in the fingers and toes, wrists and ankles. Test vibratory response with a tuning fork held over bony prominences. Test pain with pin pricks following the dermatomal pattern. Any preserved sensation or motor function below the lesion level is indicative of an incomplete injury.

Reflex activity may be absent initially, due to spinal shock (the temporary suppression of reflexes mediated below the level of injury). Reflexes return at varying time intervals, from hours to days; therefore, conduct the tests at regular intervals during the acute phase to determine when the responses begin and the type of responses elicited.

Test the bulbocavernosus reflex during a digital rectal examination by pinching the glans or base of the penis or by tugging on the Foley catheter. Involuntary contraction of the rectal sphincter during any of these maneuvers indicates a positive reflex. This implies no physiological connection between the lower spinal cord and the supraspinal centers and is indicative of a complete injury. A voluntary contraction of the sphincter during a digital rectal examination and/or rectal sensation implies continuity with the supraspinal centers, and the prognosis for further motor and sensory recovery is favorable.

The deep tendon reflexes (and their corresponding levels of innervation) most commonly tested are the biceps (C_6), triceps (C_7), quadriceps (L_{3-4}), and gastrocnemius (S_1). A positive Babinski sign (with great toe and ankle dorsiflexion, fanning of the other toes, and hip and knee flexion following plantar stimulation) is indicative of more extensive spinal cord involvement.

Radiographic Examinations

Roentgenograms can provide a means of determining the type of degree of vertebral displacement; however, knowledgeable supervision by a physician is essential, to avoid any movements that

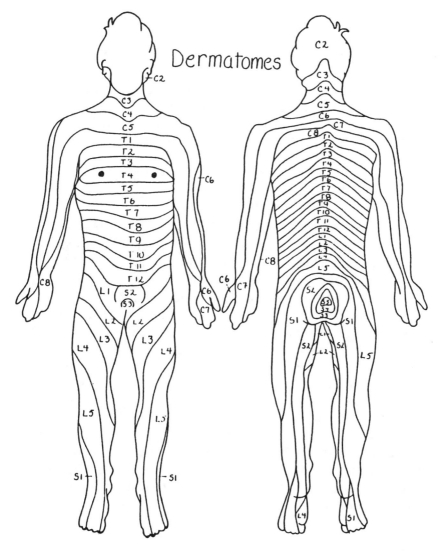

Figure 4.1 Dermatome map.

may compromise the spinal cord further. The motor and sensory examinations usually are more significant than X-ray films, as the extent of bony displacement at the moment of injury may not be evident following initial stabilization measures. A myelogram is another type of radiographic study that may be performed. Radiopaque dye is injected into the spinal subarachnoid space through a lumbar puncture needle. Distortions of the spinal cord caused by bone or foreign bodies then can be visualized. Risks of this procedure include a possible reaction to the dye resulting in headache and nausea.

Computerized axial tomography (CAT scan) is a non-invasive procedure that provides a more precise visualization of vertebral fractures and dislocations than standard X-rays. Magnetic resonance imaging (MRI) demonstrates cord compression and hemorrhage.

Electric Stimulation Test

SEPs (somatosensory evoked potentials) provide more sophisticated means of diagnostic study. Electrodes connected to a special monitor are attached to the patient's head. The peripheral nerves in the upper and lower extremities then are stimulated. If there is any continuity between these nerves and the supraspinal centers, the response will be recorded on the monitor. This study has proved to be a useful and reliable prognostic indicator.

TREATMENT OF
SPINAL CORD INJURY

As indicated in Chapter 2, treatments to minimize or reverse spinal cord damage are largely experimental at this time. The most widely accepted treatment currently in use seems to be the administration of a seven- to ten-day course of glucocorticoids to reduce spinal cord edema.

VERTEBRAL-COLUMN
STABILIZATION

Internal Procedures

Depending on the results of the diagnostic studies the physician may decide on surgical treatment. A laminectomy (removal of vertebral arch) may be done for evaluation and/or to remove the cause of pressure on the cord, such as a bone fragment or a bullet.

An anterior (Cloward) or posterior fusion may be done to immobilize the cervical spine if external stabilizing measures have not maintained alignment effectively. This also may be done to shorten the amount of time the patient must remain immobilized. Fractures of the thoracic spine often are stable because of the supporting trunk musculature and so may not require surgical intervention. For unstable thoracolumbar fractures, distraction and compression instrumentation are the procedures of choice. Postoperative care of any patient with spinal surgery is focused on accurate assessment and reporting, maintaining spinal alignment, and preventing the complications to be discussed in succeeding chapters.

Take neurological vital signs as frequently as the patient's condition warrants. Check surgical dressings at regular intervals. If a Hemovac® is present, measure and record the specific amount and quality of drainage. If the patient has a cervical injury, assess for and report any increasing sore throat, difficulty in swallowing and/or stridor, as these symptoms may be indicative of laryngeal swelling and potential airway obstruction.

Set up a regular turning schedule based on the patient's medical and skin tolerance requirements. If he has cervical traction, keep the rope and weights free and in alignment with the long axis of the cervical spine at all times. When turning him, maintain spinal alignment by moving his head and body as one unit. Turn the patient who has a thoracic or lumbar fracture in the same coordinated manner to maintain spinal alignment. When the patient is on his side, support his top leg on pillows to avoid any motion that might put strain on the spinal column.

External Alignment Devices

External stabilizing devices may be used following spinal surgery or in place of surgery. To maintain thoracic and lumbar alignment the following devices may be used.

1. A Jewett brace provides spinal column extension by means of a metal frame with vinyl padding which fits over the sternum, symphysis pubis, and small of the back (see Figure 4.2).

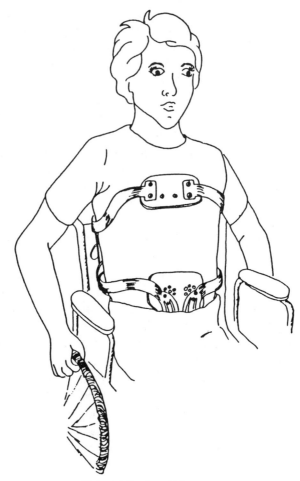

Figure 4.2   Jewett brace.

2. A molded two-part plastic jacket also may be used to provide external stabilization.

To maintain cervical alignment any of the following may be
used.

1. A Guilford brace consists of rigid struts between a chest
   plate and chin support anteriorly and between a back
   plate and occipital support posteriorly with leather straps
   connecting the anterior and posterior sections.

2. A Minerva Jacket is a molded plastic jacket providing firm support to the neck. It extends from the back of the head to hips with detachable front section from chin to hips.

3. A Philadelphia collar is a two-piece molded plastic collar for providing neck support and maintaining neck alignment.

4. Soft (foam) collars may be used for muscle support when vertebral stabilization has been assured.

5. A SOMI brace (sternal occipital mandibular immobilization) consists of metal supports connected to vinyl padding for each supported area.

In addition to these four, one of the most widely used external cervical stabilizing devices is the halo (see Figure 4.3). A chief advantage of the halo over other types of stabilization methods is that it makes early mobilization possible without compromising spinal alignment. Halo designs vary, but the basic components include a steel ring, two occipital and two temporal screws, steel bars that connect the ring to a plastic or plaster vest, and the vest itself.

The following steps provide an overview of a two-person halo application procedure. Obtain more specific instructions from the individual manufacturer.

1. Explain the purpose of the halo and its application procedure to the patient.

2. Assemble the halo components, positioning plates, supplies for pin insertion, wrenches, torque screwdriver, and tape measure.

3. Hold patient's head and neck in alignment while measurements are made for ring size. Place ring one cm above bridge of nose, using positioning plates to achieve a 1.5-cm clearance on all sides.

4. Select two temporal pin sites one cm above lateral third of eyebrows, and two occipital pin sites one cm above top of ears. Remove ring and cleanse sites with antiseptic solution.

5. Replace ring and hold in place with positioning plates and pins. Inject pin sites with local anesthetic. Put on sterile gloves.

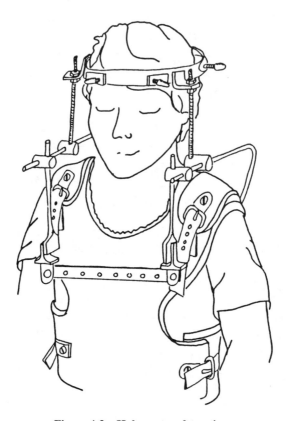

Figure 4.3   Halo vest and traction.

6. Insert pins at 90° angle to skull. Tighten pins with torque screwdriver to 2.5 kg to force and put lock-nut over each pin.

7. Position sheepskin-lined anterior and posterior vest portions on patient and loosely attach metal bars.

8. Tighten bolts connecting metal bars to ring to achieve adequate degree of traction.

9. Verify vertebral alignment with roentgenograms; recheck all component connecting bolts for tightness; buckle vest straps before moving patient. Tape correct size wrench to anterior vest for use in emergency.

The following guidelines outline the ongoing management considerations for the patient in a halo.

1. Cleanse pin sites twice daily with a disinfectant solution and normal saline. Report any drainage, inflammation, pain, increased temperature, or headache immediately.

2. Check pins periodically to insure proper tightness. Persistent loosening of screws may result from an insertion-site infection or ill-fitting vest.

3. Check skin under the vest and turn the patient frequently. If not medically contraindicated, the prone position is very beneficial, as it takes pressure off the scapula, aids in skin inspection, and aids in preventing stasis-induced respiratory, gastrointestinal, and urinary complications.

4. Never move the patient by pulling on the bars or the vest. Both actions place a strain on the metal hardware, which could affect cervical alignment.

5. Check screws daily to insure adequate tightness.

6. If cardiac resuscitation is needed, lift the anterior vest according to manufacturer's instructions.

7. If two intubation attempts are unsuccessful during a respiratory arrest, a tracheostomy is usually the procedure of choice.

Cervical Traction

Four types of tongs in common use are the Crutchfield (see Figure 4.4), the Vinke, the Gardner Wells, and the Cone Barton.

Prior to insertion of the tongs, explain the procedure to the patient. Then cleanse the insertion sites with an antiseptic solution and inject them with a local anesthetic. Burr holes are made in the outer table of the skull and the tongs are inserted. Traction weights then are added in the amount necessary to achieve reduction of the dislocation and maintain alignment.

The following are very general guidelines related to cervical traction management.

1. Clean tong insertion sites twice daily with a disinfectant solution and normal saline. Report immediately any drainage, inflammation, pain, increased temperature, or headache.

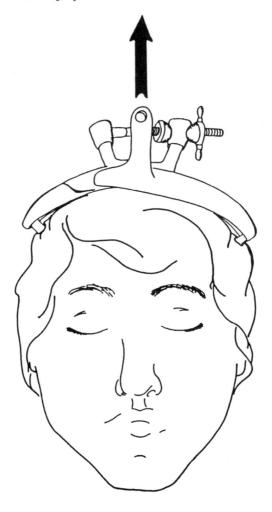

Figure 4.4   Crutchfield tongs.

2. Always keep traction ropes and weights free and in alignment with the long axis of the cervical spine.
3. Turn patient by logrolling or by using a special turning
   frame.

TURNING FRAMES

Two of the most commonly used manually operated turning
frames are the Stryker Wedge® and the Foster Frame®. Both

types have anterior and posterior frames that attach to the turning structure. After the patient has been secured safely between the two frames, the device is turned by pulling on the turning lever. After the turn, the upper frame is removed.

The Roto-Rest® and Stoke-Eggerton are electrically powered beds that turn the patient side to side. As with the manually operated turning frame, equipment must be checked for safety and traction ropes and weights must be kept free and in alignment with the spine. These beds offer several physiological advantages in addition to pressure relief on the skin, namely, continuous postural drainage and improved circulation and kidney drainage.

Because there are multiple systemic effects following any spinal cord trauma, many diagnostic and management procedures will be performed concurrently, as the following chapters will explain.

5

CARDIOVASCULAR CONSIDERATIONS

PHYSIOLOGY OVERVIEW

The circulatory system, composed of the heart, arteries, arterioles, capillaries, venules, veins, and blood has numerous functions: (1) transporting oxygen and nutrients to the cells, (2) carrying carbon dioxide and waste products away from the cells, (3) carrying hormones to their destinations, (4) assisting in the maintenance of acid-base and fluid balance, and (5) assisting in fighting disease.

Effective performance of these functions is dependent on coronary blood flow, the strength and rate of the cardiac pumping action, peripheral resistance, and blood volume and viscosity.

Vasomotor Center Activity

The vasomotor center in the medullary portion of the brainstem controls, through the autonomic nervous system, the degree of vasoconstriction, and vasodilation and the heart rate. The medulla also contains the respiratory center. The cardiovascular and respiratory actions are necessarily interrelated and interdependent. Sympathetic impulses increase the rate of the heart and the strength of contraction, thus increasing arterial pressure. The sympathetic impulses also cause peripheral vasoconstriction, further increasing the arterial pressure. Conversely, parasympathetic impulses decrease cardiac activity but have a minimal influence on the peripheral circulation.

Chemoreceptors. Stimulation of the vasomotor center can be achieved by a reflex feedback system. Changes in blood chemistry are balanced by chemoreceptors in the medulla, carotid sinus, and aortic arch. These receptor cells are particularly sensitive to elevations of circulating carbon dioxide and can catalyze the compensatory response. Medullary ischemia also stimulates the vasomotor center to send sympathetic impulses. Both chemical stimuli result in a reestablishment of the carbon dioxide-oxygen balance.

Baroreceptors. Inhibition of the vasomotor center is achieved by impulses from baroreceptors (pressoreceptors). These baroreceptors, located in the aortic arch and in the carotid sinus, detect the degree of arterial wall pressure. The greater the pressure the more impulses they send, causing vasodilation and lowered blood pressure. When the pressure falls too low, they lose their stimulation and the vasomotor center becomes excessively stimulated to send more vasoconstrictive impulses.

Venous Return

The return of venous blood to the heart is facilitated by respiratory and skeletal muscle activity. On inspiration the diaphragm contracts; the thoracic cavity enlarges; and the abdominal cavity is compressed. Correspondingly, pressure on the thoracic vessels decreases, pressure on the abdominal vessels increases, and venous return is promoted. When skeletal muscles contract they milk the blood in the veins upward toward the heart. When the muscle relaxes, the blood is kept from moving back by the semilunar valves in the veins.

VASOMOTOR SHOCK

Disruption of the autonomic nervous system innervation following a spinal cord injury results in cardiovascular manifestations. The injured person experiences profound hypotension and bradycardia from loss of sympathetic impulses. This condition is termed *vasomotor (neurogenic) shock*. It is essential that a differential diagnosis be made between vasomotor and hypovolemic shock, as the management is very different. The large quantity of blood lost in hypovolemic shock results in hypotension, tachycardia, and cool, clammy skin. To treat, one must stop the excess bleeding and replace fluid volume. Since the hypotension seen in vasomotor shock is not a result of fluid loss, pulmonary edema and congestive heart failure could be precipitated if the amount of parenteral fluid administered were not carefully controlled. The recommended parameters for parental fluid administration are based on the patient's response. Regulate the amount of fluid to achieve a systolic pressure of 100 mg Hg and to maintain a minimum hourly urine output of 25 to 30 cc.

While the importance of differentiating between vasomotor and hypovolemic shock has been stressed, this can be difficult, as many traumatic injuries may have both conditions present at the same time. In such cases, consider the management guidelines for both concomitantly; that is, treat hypovolemia with fluid replacement, but within the realm of safety to prevent fluid overload (using 100 mg Hg as the systolic parameter).

CARDIAC IRREGULARITIES AND SINUS ARREST

Cardiac irregularities and arrests may be triggered by excess vagal stimulation and hypoxia, particularly following tracheal suctioning, and by hypokalemia. During the first seven to 10 days following injury, maintain the patient on a cardiac monitor and perform frequent electrolyte determinations. Atropine® may be ordered or a pacemaker inserted if dangerous cardiac slowing occurs. Oxygenate the patient well before each suctioning period and stop the procedure immediately if any adverse change occurs in cardiac rate and rhythm.

THROMBOPHLEBITIS AND PULMONARY EMBOLISM

Other serious cardiovascular complications commonly seen during the acute stage following injury are thrombophlebitis and pulmonary embolism. A number of causative factors may be involved: (1) venous stasis secondary to paralysis of abdominal and lower-extremity muscles and general immobility, (2) hypercoagulability secondary to surgery or trauma, and (3) vessel wall damage secondary to excess pressure or trauma.

Thrombophlebitis

Due to the patient's sensory loss the first sign of phlebitis may be a noticeable asymmetry of the involved lower extremity, rather than pain. Diagnosis would be confirmed with phlebography showing a thrombus and lack of venous filling, increased areas of radioactivity on a fibrinogen scan, or continuous blood flow with no respiratory modulations during Doppler studies.

To treat thrombophlebitis, improve blood flow with bed rest, elevation of the extremity, and elastic support stockings; and prevent hypercoagulability with anticoagulant drugs. Fibrinolytic drugs also may be administered.

Pulmonary Embolism

Initial symptoms of pulmonary embolism may be multiple and inconclusive, such as anxiety, dyspnea, tachycardia, hypotension, diaphoresis, hemoptysis, and fever. More specific diagnostic indicators include a pleural friction rub, an elevated lactic dehydrogenase (LDH) level, visualization of filling defects on a pulmonary angiogram, areas of increased radioactivity on a lung scan, an enlarged P wave and other characteristic changes on an electrocardiogram, and blood gases showing low pO_2 and low pCO_2. To treat pulmonary embolism, administer anticoagulants; relieve hypoxemia with oxygen administration; and relieve pain, anxiety, and other symptoms with appropriate measures.

Preventive Measures

To prevent both conditions, employ the following measures: (1) use properly fitted elastic support stockings and/or herring-boned ace wraps, (2) encourage a daily range of motion and early mobilization, (3) position patient to avoid pressure over large vessels, (4) encourage deep breathing exercises, (5) ensure adequate fluid intake, and (6) maintain proper intravenous management. Very small doses (5000 μ) of heparin twice daily can be utilized as a more aggressive prophylactic approach until the patient is fully mobilized.

ORTHOSTATIC HYPOTENSION AND LOWER-EXTREMITY EDEMA

As discussed previously, sympathetic effects help maintain blood pressure through vasoconstriction, and the abdominal and lower-extremity muscles facilitate venous return through their alternating compressive actions. Depending on the amount of sympathetic disruption and skeletal muscle paralysis following an SCI, there will be varying degrees of orthostatic hypotension and lower-extremity edema.

To minimize these adverse effects, the SCI patient should wear an abdominal binder and elastic support stockings. Move him slowly from a lying to a sitting position. Initially, provide him with a reclining wheelchair with elevating footrests. A progressive tilting schedule on a specially designed board also may be helpful in facilitating upright tolerance for the newly injured patient. When he has regained a functional degree of vasomotor stability, the binder, elastic support stockings, reclining wheelchair, and tilt table may be eliminated.

SUMMARY

During the acute stage following an SCI, the patient is likely to develop cardiovascular complications as a result of autonomic nervous system disruption, electrolyte imbalances, and immobility. With time, increased mobility, and preventive management, his cardiovascular homeostasis will be restored; and with adequate knowledge and compliance he can maintain this balance. However, with the aging process other cardiovascular problems begin to emerge such as hypertension and coronary artery disease. As with the general population, preventive teaching and early intervention are of crucial importance in reducing morbidity and mortality rates.

6

RESPIRATORY MANAGEMENT

ANATOMY AND PHYSIOLOGY

Ventilation is a cyclic process of moving oxygenated air into the lungs (inspiration) and removing carbon dioxide (expiration). The respiratory center in the medulla oblongata controls the rate and depth of ventilations. Any increase in the arterial blood level of carbon dioxide or decrease in arterial oxygen is detected by chemoreceptors located in the aortic arch, carotid arteries, and medulla. These receptors stimulate the respiratory center, which then sends impulses down the spinal cord via the phrenic and intercostal nerves to the diaphragm and intercostal muscles.

Inspiration occurs when the contraction of these muscles expands the thoracic cavity and decreases intrapulmonic pressure. Atmospheric air is then drawn through the nose, pharynx, larynx, and tracheobronchial tree to the alveoli to equalize this negative pressure.

Expiration occurs as the inspiratory muscles relax, reducing the size of the thoracic cavity and increasing intrapulmonic pressure. This increased pressure pushes air out of the lungs until the intrapulmonic and atmospheric pressure are again equalized. Coughing, a forced expiration, is achieved by a sudden contraction of the abdominal muscles.

Perfusion refers to the process that supplies the lung capillaries with blood from the right side of the heart. It requires an adequate cardiac pumping action, patent blood vessels, and sufficient blood volume. Diffusion, the exchange of oxygen and carbon dioxide, occurs in the alveoli and the capillaries. It requires adequate ventilatory function to transport the air to and from the alveoli. Respiration refers to the entire process of gas exchange within the lungs and between the cells and the blood. In addition to adequately functioning cardiovascular and ventilatory systems, a sufficient amount of hemoglobin is needed in the blood to combine with and transport the oxygen molecules to the cells.

RESPIRATORY EFFECTS OF
SPINAL CORD INJURY

Those injuries at C_4 or above will have phrenic nerve damage with partial or complete diaphragm paralysis. Injuries between T_2–T_{12} affect the intercostal muscles and the individual's ability to deep breathe effectively. Injuries between T_6–T_{12} can paralyze the abdominal muscles and the individual's ability to forcefully exhale and cough.

Pneumothorax and respiratory fatigue are two of the problems that may occur during the initial days following injury in any person with a high thoracic or cervical lesion. Ascending spinal cord edema is a potential danger, as it may compromise further or even abolish the remaining intercostal or diaphragm function.

Gastric distension, resulting from autonomic disruption, also can restrict or abolish diaphragmatic motion (see Chapter 9). Pulmonary edema is another condition that could compromise respiratory function further. It can occur as a result of excess parenteral fluid administration during vasomotor shock management (see Chapter 5).

Inability to clear secretions effectively results from partial or complete paralysis of the inspiratory and expiratory muscles (lesions above T_{12}). This can lead to atelectasis, pneumonia, and acute bronchial obstruction by mucus plugs. These complications further reduce ventilatory efficiency by blocking air exchange in various parts of the lung.

DIAGNOSTIC TESTS

After the newly injured individual has been brought to the hospital, conduct diagnostic tests to clarify his respiratory status and to determine the appropriate support measures that will be needed for on-going management. Obtain a chest X-ray, an abdominal flat plate, and vital capacity measurements with a Wright respirometer or incentive spirometer. Arterial blood gases also should be drawn to obtain baseline values.

Continue to monitor the patient frequently to detect any significant changes in respiratory rate and quality, as well as any changes in vital capacity, vital signs, and blood gases. Such changes could warn of atelectasis, respiratory infection, hemopneumothorax, pulmonary embolism, or impending diaphragm fatigue.

When the patient has stabilized medically, perform pulmonary function studies to assess the extent of respiratory impairment and to evaluate the effectiveness of treatment regimes. The tidal volume in the quadriplegic patient usually will be within the normal range, and the other values will be greatly decreased, except for the residual volume. This is markedly increased, due to paralysis of the muscles of expiration; thus he is more prone to develop congestion and often will have a lowered PaO_2 and elevated PCO_2.

His vital capacity will vary according to his position. It is reduced when he sits, as his paralyzed abdominal muscles allow gravity to pull the viscera and diaphragm lower in the abdominal cavity. This problem can be overcome partially by the use of an abdominal binder to support the abdominal wall. He will have an increased vital capacity in a Trendelenburg position as the weight of the viscera pushes his diaphragm higher on expiration. This then allows for greater diaphragmatic excursion on inspiration.

PREVENTION GUIDELINES

Because of the compromised or absent abilities to cough and deep breathe effectively, and because of the general immobility imposed by the injury, a spinal cord patient is prone to develop atelectasis and pneumonia. To prevent these complications, include the following measures in his ongoing treatment plan (frequency of each is determined by his current status):

1. Turning and deep breathing exercises using an incentive spirometer
2. Percussion (rhythmic, gentle clapping over congested areas with hands in cupped position)
3. Vibration (manual compression and tremor to chest wall during exhalation)

4. Assistive coughing (firm pressure applied in and upward beneath diaphragm during forceful expiration)
5. Postural drainage (gravity assisted drainage with congested area in uppermost position)

An intermittent positive pressure breathing (IPPB) machine also may be used to increase alveolar ventilation by supplying air or oxygen under increased pressure during inspiration. Bronchodilator or mucolytic agents may be administered during the treatment (vital signs should be checked before and after initial use of bronchodilator). The machine's pressure gauge usually is set at 15–20 cm H_2O. A slight inspiration by the patient should be sufficient to activate the positive pressure phase. A closed circuit (no nose breathing) is necessary for treatment to be effective.

TRACHEOSTOMY CARE

Some patients, as a result of the previously discussed complications, may need to be intubated or have a tracheostomy performed. (Refer to your institution's policies and procedures for endotracheal tube management and pre- and postoperative tracheostomy management.)

The two types of tubes most frequently used with a tracheostomy are: a cuffless metal tube with an outer and inner cannula and a cuffed tube with an outer and inner cannula and a pilot balloon to keep the internal cuff inflated. A cuffed trach is preferred for initial management, especially for ventilator dependent patients since the cuff provides a greater seal. For chronic management, the metal trach is preferred because of its low risk for tracheal necrosis.

Special attention must be directed toward supplying adequate humidification to the respiratory passages with any type of tracheostomy tube, to prevent dehydrated mucosa and viscous secretions.

Suctioning

Suctioning any SCI patient can be hazardous; vagal stimulation may decrease heart rate further to the point of sinus arrest, and pulling oxygen out may exacerbate a hypoxic condition and potentiate cardiac arrhythmias. Therefore, suction only when necessary following these guidelines:

1. Assemble equipment.
2. Place patient in sitting position if not contraindicated.
3. Ventilate with 80–100% of oxygen concentration for three to five minutes.
4. Attach catheter (size less than half of diameter of tracheostomy tube) to connecting tube and turn on suction (-80 to -120 mm Hg pressure).
5. With gloved hand lubricate patient end of catheter, then gently insert eight to 12 in. (unoccluded) into tracheostomy.
6. For tenacious secretions use a syringe with needle removed and instill three to five ml sterile normal saline.
7. To aspirate right bronchus, instruct patient to turn head to left; then elevate his chin (if not contraindicated neurologically) and tilt chest to right. Use opposite directions for left bronchus.
8. Occlude thumb control, suction by rotating catheter while withdrawing (10 s maximum).
9. Rinse catheter with sterile water, oxygenate patient, and repeat suctioning as needed.
10. Be alert for possible bradycardia, tachycardia, or arrythmias. Remove catheter immediately and oxygenate if any occur.
11. Reoxygenate patient after procedure.

Care of Equipment

While stoma care, cuff pressure measurements, and inner cannula care are performed according to individual hospital procedures, the requirements of the specific patient, and the type of tracheostomy tube used, the following general guidelines may be useful.
Inner Cannula Care.

1. Elevate head of bed 45° if not contraindicated.
2. Oxygenate and suction patient.

3. Wearing gloves, remove inner cannula and soak in hydrogen peroxide and cold water.
4. Cleanse area around stoma with normal saline.
5. Clean inner cannula with tracheostomy brush or pipe cleaners.
6. Rinse with sterile water, reinsert, and lock in place.

General Cuff Care.

1. Keep inflated when patient is being ventilated, receiving IPPB treatments, eating, or drinking.
2. Deflate when tracheostomy is plugged or when weaning from ventilator, or periodically to prevent tracheal necrosis.
3. Suction tube and oropharynx prior to each deflation.
4. Suspect a tracheo-esophageal fistula or an underinflated or ruptured cuff if an air leak is noted, if methylene blue test is positive, or if patient coughs during swallowing.

MECHANICAL VENTILATION

The patient unable to breathe independently or one who is developing increasing diaphragmatic fatigue with other signs of respiratory distress needs mechanical ventilation. Ventilators are classified as volume-cycled, pressure-cycled, or time-cycled. All push air into the patient's lungs under positive pressure. A volume-cycled ventilator ends inspiration when a preset volume has been reached. A pressure-cycled ventilator ends inspiration when a preset pressure has been reached. A time-cycled model ends respiration when a preset time interval has been reached. Expiration may be passive or against positive pressure (known as "PEEP" or "positive end expiratory pressure").

Preparation and Maintenance

Before beginning mechanical ventilation, explain the equipment, the purpose, and related procedures to the patient and his family. Evaluate his physiological parameters to determine the appropriate type of ventilator and the settings (tidal volume, pressure limit, peak flow, respiratory rate, oxygen concentration). Establish an appropriate airway; adjust machine settings; and fill the humidifier before connecting the patient.

While he is on the ventilator perform frequent assessments of his vital signs, blood gases, intake and output, and his general status (is he in respiratory or mental distress; what is his skin color and turgor; is his chest rising and falling synchronously with the ventilator; is he fighting the machine; is he in a position that facilitates breathing?).

Perform other procedures as needed, for example, suctioning, mouth care, chest therapy, and repositioning. Check equipment often to assure proper functioning, and keep manual ventilator available at all times.

Potential Complications

Because of the constant positive intrapulmonary pressure that is created by a mechanical ventilator, tension pneumothorax is a potential complication. There is also increased pressure on the great thoracic vessels, with a subsequent decrease of blood return to the heart. This will lead to a drop in blood pressure, a rise in central venous pressure, and the possible development of interstitial edema. Heart rate changes may indicate inadequate oxygenation, a compensatory response to the vascular pressure, infection, pain, and/or anxiety. Other potential complications include tracheal damage from endotracheal or tracheostomy tube pressure, oxygen toxicity from administering too high a concentration, and respiratory alkalosis from too high a respiratory rate setting.

To determine a patient's readiness for weaning, consider the following physiological parameters: pO_2 of at least 70 on a FiO_2 of 50% or less, a vital capacity of at least 15 ml per Kg, a respiratory rate between 12 and 20, and adequate muscle function to support ventilation. Prepare him prior to weaning and provide continuous emotional support during the process, as he probably will be extremely frightened.

Intermittent mandatory ventilation (IMV) often is used as an intermediate stage between controlled and spontaneous ventilation. This provides a set rate and volume lower than the previous controlled setting so the patient can breathe on his own but still receive enough assistance to give him psychological and physical support.

After IMV he usually will be put on a T-piece (a special tracheostomy adapter for supplying humidified oxygen). With this he will no longer be receiving any mechanical respiratory assistance. Patients at risk for atelectasis or congestion may benefit from PEEP during this intermediate stage.

Whatever type of weaning method is used, continue to monitor the patient closely for signs of impending problems, such as a respiratory rate increased by more than 10 per min., an apical pulse increased by more than 20 beats per min., and a blood pressure elevation of 20 mm Hg systolic and 10 mm Hg diastolic.

VENTILATOR ALTERNATIVES

The patient with an injury at C_3 or above is usually ventilator dependent. A few individuals in this category may be able to breathe on their own for short periods of time by using the accessory muscles of respiration (the sternomastoid and scalene) and by using the mouth and throat to force air into the lungs (glossopharyngeal breathing). However, these types of breathing are too fatiguing to be used on a long-term basis.

A surgically implanted phrenic nerve stimulator may be a feasible alternative to ventilator dependence for some individuals with high-level lesions. Electrodes are implanted surgically, bilaterally over the phrenic nerve innervation to the diaphragm. About two weeks after the surgery an external transmitter is activated to stimulate the electrodes and nerve. The individual may tolerate only five minutes of stimulation initially but ultimately progress to a 12-hour tolerance.

The pneumobelt may be a feasible option for the patient who is off the ventilator either temporarily or permanently, but fatigues easily or cannot maintain proper respiration in a seated position. The pneumobelt is a corset with an inflatable bladder which is attached to a portable ventilator. As the bladder inflates with air, it compresses the abdomen for the expiratory phase of respiration. As the bladder deflates, the diaphragm drops to allow for passive inspiration.

Perform frequent assessments to assure adequate equipment

functioning. Keep a manual ventilator available at all times. For further information on the care of persons who are ventilator dependent and for those who use ventilator alternatives refer to the bibliography.

SUMMARY

In the acute stage following SCI, preventive respiratory management is a primary focus. As the patient becomes more mobilized the emphasis on this area may decrease; however, it must remain a life-long concern for individuals with high cervical injuries. Receiving comprehensible information on how to maintain respiratory health not only will decrease the patient's fears but will increase his potential for an improved quality of life.

7

NUTRITIONAL CONSIDERATIONS

A daily program of balanced nutrition is essential to maintaining general good health. Physical and emotional traumas may have a disruptive influence on this nutritional balance. Nutritional imbalances also can cause or exacerbate medical problems. Review of the abundant literature on nutrition shows many conflicting opinions and studies. Despite the conflicts and unanswered questions, there remains a large body of vitally important information that must be incorporated into any medical management program.

Protein, the underlying structure of all body parts, is required for tissue formation and maintenance. Any stress on the body, such as a draining wound losing serous exudate, will increase the need for protein. The protein requirement also fluctuates with age: the younger person who is growing needs additional protein. Fat is used to store and transport other substances and to provide energy. Carbohydrates are also energy-producing foods. Vitamins, minerals, and fluid made up the remainder of the diet.

MINERALS AND VITAMINS

Because each individual's nutritional requirements depend on so many variables, it is best to consult a nutrition table for the RDA (Recommended Dietary Allowances) and calculate the needs based on the relevant variables. Although minerals take up relatively little body volume, their functions are critical and complex. Sodium, potassium, and chloride provide both positive and negative ions which permit fluid exchanges and balances within the body. Calcium, phosphorus, zinc, magnesium, and iron are the most plentiful; however, many other trace elements also can be found in the body. Vitamins are very important in many areas of metabolism and cell growth. Tables 7.1, 7.2, and 7.3 describe

TABLE 7.1 Dietary Minerals.

Mineral	Food Source	Function and SCI Implication	Miscellaneous
Calcium	Dairy products Collard and kale	Together with phosphorus, the most plentiful of the body's minerals. Necessary for contraction/relaxation of muscles; assists in clotting. Excessive protein intake decreases the utilization of calcium especially when calcium intake is limited. Vitamin D is critical for calcium use.	Calcium is bound by fat in the intestines; also bound by oxalic acid and fiber rendering it insoluble.
Phosphorus	Dairy products, meats, unprocessed foods, beans	Functions with calcium.	
Zinc	Animal food sources (most readily absorbed), seafood, nuts, whole grains	Biochemical component of enzymatic reactions. Indirect role in DNA synthesis. Integral for tissue growth and repair. Zinc levels change dramatically in response to stress, disease.	With deficiency, wounds heal slowly. Vegetarians must be careful to obtain adequate amounts. Sources of zinc may vary depending on where the food is grown.
Iron	Liver, yeast, wheat germ, egg yolks, whole grains, beans, spinach	Essential for transport of oxygen. Iron can be recycled within the body. Vitamin C and calcium enhance absorption. Iron content varies depending on where the food is grown.	Most common deficiency. Also ingested through cooking in iron pans.
Magnesium	Fruit, grains, green leafy vegetables	Important in activating enzymes, especially for protein synthesis and transfer of energy. One-half of the body's magnesium is found in the bones.	Deficiencies in magnesium generally accompany protein deficiencies and diabetes.

TABLE 7.2 Water-Soluble Vitamins

Vitamin	Food Sources	Function	Deficiency and Precautions
C Ascorbic Acid	Vegetables (broccoli, brussels sprouts, leafy greens), horseradish, fruits (mango, orange, grapefruit, cantaloupe)	Increases iron absorption and folic acid metabolism. Hastens wound healing. Transports oxygen. Participates in formation of collagen. Acts to combat infections although its role is unclear. Needs will increase with any source of stress. Necessary for energy release. Raw fish and tea antagonize thiamine. All B vitamins are synergistic. Are not easily stored so intake must be frequent. Daily requirements depend on energy needs.	Deficiency: scurvy, weakening of collagen, and delayed wound healing. Heat labile (prolonged cooking destroys Vitamin C). Can interfere with anticoagulant therapy. Cigarettes and birth control pills lower plasma Vitamin C.
Thiamine (B_1)	Wheat germ, rice polish, cereals, grains, nuts, beans	Necessary for energy release and protein synthesis. Contributes to health of skin and eyes.	Although rare in U.S., nervous system and cardiovascular system changes occur with deficiency.
Riboflavin (B_2)	Dairy products, collard greens, broccoli, yeast, beans, liver	Necessary for energy release and protein synthesis. Contributes to health of skin and eyes.	Deficiency: causes light sensitivity, purple tongue, and bloodshot eyes.
Folacin	Liver, beans, leafy vegetables, fruit	Is required for the formation of nucleic acids, synthesis and breakdown of amino acids.	Folacin is heat sensitive and is therefore destroyed by cooking.

Biotin	Functions in the metabolism of fat and carbohydrates. Synthesized by intestinal flora.	Deficiency causes anorexia, nausea, vomiting, depression, dry scaly dermatitis.
Pantothenic Acid	Important for release of energy from carbohydrates. Decreased pantothenic acid contributes to adrenal gland damage causing diminished adrenal hormone output. Stress increases the need for these hormones.	Heat unstable. Daily requirement fluctuates with stress. Deficiency results in hypoglycemia, dizziness, weakness.
Niacin	Necessary for energy release. Can sometimes be synthesized by intestinal flora. Also contributes to healthy skin. Aids in digestion.	Deficiency results in tissue damage particularly of the skin, digestive tract and nervous system.
B_6	Important for protein metabolism (e.g., red blood cell production, glucose for muscle tissue and functioning of nervous tissue). Helps maintain normal magnesium level.	Deficiency results in depression, confusion, anemia, dermatitis, elevated white blood cells. B_6 deficiency: oxalic kidney stones. B_6 and magnesium deficiency: calcium and phosphorus, kidney stones.
B_{12}	Important in its role in the synthesis of DNA and RNA and cell division. Synthesized also from intestinal flora.	Severe deficiency can cause central nervous system damage. Pernicious anemia (malabsorption of B_{12}).
Dairy products (animal sources only)		

TABLE 7.3 Fat-Soluble Vitamins

Vitamin	Food Source	Function and SCI Implications	Miscellaneous
A	Liver, fish-lever oils, egg yolks, butter and cream, carrots, hubbard and butternut squash, dandelion greens, cantaloupes, kale	Vitamin A has a variety of functions: Eyes: visual acuity, maintains epithelium; Skin: prevents pores from becoming blocked with dead cells; Nails: prevents peeling and ridging; Bones: enhances growth; Hair: responsible for sheen; Mucous membranes: maintains fatty membrane responsible for blocking out infections.	Deficiency results in night blindness. Bright light and O_2 destroy A. Must get A from both animal and vegetable sources. Toxicity can result from animal sources.
D	Most absorption occurs not from food sources but a D-precursor. This Pro-vitamin is converted to D by exposure to the sun. Milk is generally Vitamin D fortified.	Vitamin D regulates the metabolism of calcium and phosphorus for bone mineralization by increasing their absorption.	Excess D can cause excessive calcium uptake leading to deposits throughout the body. Toxicity can also result.
E	Nuts, spinach, vegetable oils, wheat germ	Functions to prevent fatty substances from being destroyed by oxygen. Necessary for formation of every cell nucleus; therefore, Vitamin E prevents cells from disintegrating. Prevents pain and scars from burns. Is thought to melt blood clots (phlebitis).	Unstable in freezing. Toxicity unlikely.
K	Leafy green vegetables, egg yolk, milk	Necessary for clotting of blood. Partially synthesized by intestinal flora.	Antibiotic therapy attacks intestinal flora and may cause resultant deficiency. Compensate by eating yogurt.

briefly the functions of the various minerals and vitamins and their implications with regard to spinal cord injury.

NUTRITION AND
SPINAL CORD INJURY

The neurological changes, immobility, and any associated medical problems of SCI cause secondary disruptions in other body systems. Nutritional requirements fluctuate in accordance with the individual's current physiological status.

Mechanical Considerations

Mechanical problems may affect an individual's nutritional status by interfering with chewing or swallowing. If the neck is hyperextended by an orthotic device, swallowing may be difficult and frightening. General body positioning also may limit the jaw movement and interfere with chewing. Modifications in the diet, such as soft foods, may be helpful in these situations, as they are easier to swallow and require minimal chewing. Prior to a meal, position the patient in the most optimal position possible to make eating easier. Prism glasses, for the person in a halo or on a turning frame, will increase visibility.

Physiological Considerations

Gastrointestinal Changes. Paralytic ileus is a complication frequently encountered immediately after injury. Until it resolves, give the patient nothing by mouth. Should this resolution take longer than four to five days, a potentially serious nutritional imbalance may occur. Used within the bounds of cardiovascular safety, parenteral treatment may prevent further nutritional deterioration. Initiate a high-protein diet once the paralytic ileus is resolved.

Endogenous or iatric steroids and hypersecretion of hydrochloric acid may cause gastritis and ulcers. These conditions will affect the patient's appetite and tolerance for certain foods. Small, frequent, and easily digested meals may be helpful.

A negative nitrogen balance is another common result of the overproduction of adrenocortical hormones. A high-protein diet is beneficial in moderating this catabolic response.

Elimination problems also will affect the nutritional status (see Chapter 9). Make a thorough assessment of prior diet and elimination habits and current medications, diet, and mobility status. This is an important step in planning a functional bowel routine that will resolve these problems.

Genitourinary Changes. Urinary tract infections (UTI) and renal calculi are other complications that may follow an SCI and will require nutritional assessment and intervention. Encourage copious fluids when a catheter is in place and during febrile episodes, particularly those resulting from a UTI. Provide the patient with cranberry and grape juices to help acidify his urine and decrease the potential for calculi and bacteriuria. Calcium intake once was thought to contribute to stone formation and therefore was limited. In recent years the efficacy of this prophylactic approach has come into question.

Metabolic Changes. During the acute stage following injury, fluid and electrolyte balance may be altered; therefore, close monitoring is important so that the appropriate replacements can be provided and balance restored.

After the patient's medical status has stabilized, decreased mobility may result in an undesirable weight gain. Early intervention and education can prevent this problem from occurring.

Skin Changes. The presence of a decubitus increases the need for certain nutrients that are depleted rapidly when infection is present, because they play significant roles in the healing process. Sufficient protein, a major component of cellular structure, is essential for any healing to occur. Besides the standard sources, additional protein can be obtained through high-protein supplements. The need for vitamins and some minerals also increases when a decubitus is present. For example, Vitamin A helps to restore the integrity of a skin's epithelium. Vitamin C facilitates wound healing. Zinc, a trace element, also has been found to expedite wound healing by affecting cell growth and repair.

Psychosocial Considerations

Many emotional factors can affect an individual's desire to eat, such as depression, embarrassment at having to be fed, and frustration with independent feeding attempts. Therefore, being sensitive to the individual's emotional needs is an essential component of nutritional planning. Careful assessment of pre-injury patterns may be helpful in formulating postinjury diet plans. Foods and fluids that are handled easily as well as the necessary assistive devices may facilitate eating.

Cultural Background

In a thorough dietary history, include what beliefs the patient and his family hold and what implications these may have on present planning. For instance, the Italian diet, typically high in calcium and carbohydrates, may need modifications that will accommodate both the psychological and physiological needs of an Italian patient.

More subtle beliefs, such as "a healthy child is a fat child" or "eating may make you feel better" also can affect how the patient perceives and adapts to dietary changes. Include significant family members in any nutritional planning, as their understanding and cooperation may be crucial to the patient's adjustment.

8

UROLOGICAL MANAGEMENT

ANATOMY

The kidneys, composed of approximately two million delicate tubules called nephrons, produce urine. In doing so, they regulate the volume and composition of body fluids, conserve water and other essential substances, maintain an acid-base balance, and detoxify and excrete foreign, noxious, or nonessential materials. The filtrate then travels through the ureters (see Figure 8.1) to the urinary bladder, a vessel composed of smooth muscle called the detrusor. A valve at the junction of the kidneys and ureters prevents any backflow of urine to the kidneys.

PHYSIOLOGY OF MICTURITION

Micturition is under both reflex and voluntary control. The micturition reflex is initiated when the quantity of urine in the bladder stimulates intramuscular sensory fibers. These fibers then send impulses via the pelvic (parasympathetic) nerve to the sacral reflex center located at the S2 to S4 level of the spinal cord. From there the impulses continue up the spinothalamic and posterior columns to the micturition centers in the frontal cortex and brain stem. Impulses from the brain stem move down the reticulospinal tract to the pelvic nerves. The pelvic nerves stimulate detrusor contraction, closure of the ureter orifices, and internal sphincter (bladder neck) relaxation. Voluntary control, maintained by contraction and relaxation of the external sphincter and pelvic floor muscles, is regulated by impulses moving from the frontal cortex down the corticospinal tract to the pudendal nerve. Sympathetic fibers are associated with bladder filling and urine storage. Adrenergic stimulation results in contraction at the bladder neck and outlet and detrusor relaxation.

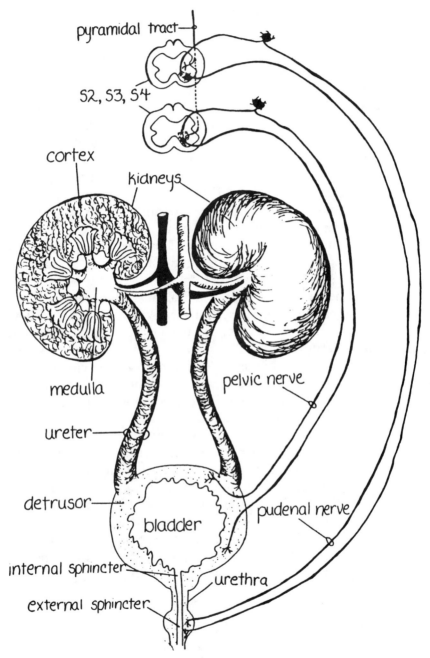

Figure 8.1 **Neurophysiology of the urinary system.**

EFFECTS OF SPINAL CORD INJURY

Spinal cord injury (SCI) can affect any part of the micturition process, depending on the location and extent of neurological damage. A neurogenic bladder is the term used to refer to these effects. The bladder management program depends largely on the neurological dysfunction that diagnostic tests illustrate.

Neurogenic bladders are categorized as to the type of dysfunction: failure to store occurs when the reflex arc is intact and results in urge, stress, or reflex incontinence. This type of neurogenic bladder is also classified as reflex hypertonic, automatic, or upper motor neuron. Failure to empty occurs when peripheral nerve damage impairs the reflex arc and results in urinary retention and overflow incontinence. This type of neurogenic bladder is also classified as autonomous, hypotonic, or lower motor neuron.

The subject of neurogenic bladder management is multidimensional involving psychological, physiological, and educational parameters. Urological dysfunction can be an embarrassing, disrupting, and isolating problem for persons with neurological disabilities. In addition to the psychological ramifications, they are susceptible to life threatening physiological complications. Therefore, patient education is essential to help them regain a sense of control and confidence as well as to maximize bladder self-care abilities and prevent complications.

The goals of a nursing management plan include helping patients achieve and maintain balanced, functional bladders free from preventable complications, helping patients cope with the stress of urological dysfunction, and assisting them in learning to successfully manage their own regimes. The interventions required to achieve these goals are determined by each individual's neurological and urological status, preexisting health problems, age, sex, psychosocial status, and discharge plan.

DIAGNOSTIC TESTS

In addition to a health history and physical assessment, a complete urologic profile will facilitate the choice of bladder routine and demonstrate any pathologic conditions. A variety of diagnostic tests may be recommended:

- Blood tests to rule out electrolyte imbalances and renal impairment
- Urodynamic studies: Cystometrics to measure bladder and sphincter tone, filling pressure, and capacity; electromyography to diagnose detrusor sphincter dyssynergy; and urethral pressure profile to identify sites of urethral resistance and to measure pressure
- Cystoscopy to determine presence of pathology through direct visualization
- Renal ultrasound to demonstrate presence of hydronephrosis, calculi, and renal
- Cystourethrogram (voiding and retrograde) to observe the shape and capacity of the bladder and to rule out pathologies such as urethral diverticulum, reflux, tumors, and calculi
- Intravenous pyelogram (see Figure 8.2) to observe upper urinary tract anatomy and to rule out renal and ureteric changes (IVP associated with high risk of renal failure in elderly)
- Renal scan to demonstrate any upper tract disturbances such as reflux and hydronephrosis
- Kidney/ureter/bladder radiograph to determine presence of calculi; to demonstrate bladder shape and presence of dilated ureters
- Renal scintigraphy and arteriography to rule out urinary tract pathology and to demonstrate renal blood flow
- Urine studies to determine presence of infection and renal impairment

METHODS OF EMPTYING A NEUROGENIC BLADDER

Failure to Store

For reflex incontinence establish an intermittent catheterization program (ICP) every 4 hours with progression dependent on catheterization volume and/or post void residuals. An ICP can main-

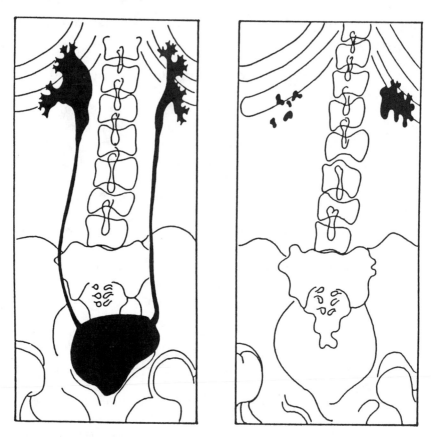

**Figure 8.2   Intravenous pyelogram demonstrating (a) hydronephrosis of the
right kidney and (b) staghorn calculus in the left kidney and multiple calculi in
the right kidney.**

tain the health of the urinary system by preventing recurrent UTIs
from urine stagnation and bladder distention, preventing kidney
damage from bladder distention and ureteral reflux, relieving the
patient of incontinence, and restoring bladder tone and function
through periodic emptying. ICP is contraindicated when fluids
cannot be restricted or in the presence of anatomical abnormali-
ties such as meatal or urethral stenosis. Employ trigger techniques
to facilitate reflex emptying in addition to ICP (or instead of ICP
when post void residuals are less than 20 percent of bladder capacity). Assist the patient in learning self-catheterization and/or
trigger techniques and fluid regulation.

Select appropriate urinary containment devices for incontinence such as condom devices and incontinence briefs. There are female external devices available but adherence and skin irritation remain major problems. Assist the patient in learning correct application, removal, and skin care techniques.

Promote storing by administering prescribed medication to increase urethral and bladder neck resistance (ephedrine/Ephedsol, phenylephrine/Sudafed); to decrease bladder contractility and spasticity (hyoscyamine sulfate/Levisin, oxybutynin chloride/Ditropan, flavoxate/Urispas, imipramine/Tofranil, hyoscyamine/Cystospaz, propantheline bromide/Pro Banthine). Observe and record patient response. Take precautions to minimize side effects of the medications. Assist the patient in learning the medication purpose, dosage, schedule, side effects, and precautions.

Failure to Empty

For urinary retention establish an ICP every 4 hours with progression dependent on catheterization volume and patient's fluid intake. Assist the patient in learning fluid regulation, self-catheterization techniques, and/or techniques to facilitate voiding (with the urologist approval) such as the Valsalva or crede maneuver or the anal sphincter stretch.

Insert an indwelling catheter only when other strategies are inappropriate as with ureteral reflux. To prevent a penoscrotal fistula or urethral diverticula, select smallest size catheter with the smallest balloon whenever possible and tape the catheter to the patient's abdomen (male) or upper thigh (female). (Note: An indwelling catheter may also be required when fluid restriction is contraindicated for the patient with incontinence.) Assist the patient in learning catheter insertion and management techniques and the importance of increased fluid intake (3000–4000 cc qd).

Promote emptying by administering prescribed medication to enhance bladder contractility (bethanecol hydrochloride/Urecholine); to increase relaxation of urethral smooth muscle and decrease outflow resistance (phenoxybenzamine/Dibenzyline, terazosin/Hytrin, prazosin/Minipress); and/or to increase relaxation of striated external sphincter (diazepam/Valium, baclofen/Lioresal, dantrolene sodium/Dantrium).

A uro-stent is a nonsurgical option that may be used to hold the urethra open.

COMPLICATIONS

Urologic complications, either acute or chronic can plague the person with SCI. Prompt and effective treatment, however, can resolve the problems. Some problems and treatments are presented in Table 8.1.

SURGICAL INTERVENTIONS

The urethral prosthesis is designed to simulate normal action of the perineum and sphincter by closing off the urethra. Two rod-shaped tubes are inserted parallel to the urethra. These rods are connected to a pressure device in the groin that allows the individual to inflate (close) and deflate (open) the prosthesis. This eliminates the daily need for catheterization. For this to be a satisfactory alternative, the individual needs to have enough upper extremity strength and dexterity to perform transfers, undress, and manipulate the prosthesis. Assist the patient in learning proper management techniques.

With the continent vesicotomy an anterior flap of the bladder wall is formed into a valve-like intussusception which leads to a stoma on the anterior abdominal wall. It is a reversible procedure. The potential complications include suture dehiscence, stomal stenosis, infection, and calculi.

Augmentation cystoplasty is a surgical procedure that enlarges the bladder by using a portion of the ileum or fundus of the stomach.

The objective of a transurethral resection and external sphincterotomy (TURES) is to diminish bladder neck and sphincter resistance to urine outflow. The criteria for surgery are based on a variety of clinical and diagnostic parameters including the presence of severe detrusor sphincter dyssynergia, vesico-ureteric reflux, high residuals with hyperreflexia, or upper tract changes with sustained high intravesical pressure and spastic sphincter. Because permanent incontinence is one result, the sphincterotomy should not be performed on anyone who has the potential for more neurological return. Assist the patient in understanding the procedure and follow-up care that is required.

Extracorporeal shock-wave lithotripsy (ESWL) uses shock waves generated outside the body to break up kidney stones inside the body without harming the kidneys or nearby organs. The advantages over traditional kidney surgery include a shorter hospital stay, reduced incidence of pain, and a decreased risk of complications. Percutaneous lithotripsy is another procedure that may be used if the patient is not a candidate for ESWL. In this procedure the kidney stones are removed through a catheter that has been introduced into the kidney collecting system through an incision over the site.

SUMMARY

Loss of bladder control can be an embarrassing, humiliating experience for most people. Helping the patient learn how to manage this aspect of his personal care successfully and independently can increase his feelings of confidence and internal control. The establishment and maintenance of a satisfactory bladder routine takes time and patience.

TABLE 8.1 Urinary Tract Complications

Pathology	Definition	Signs & Symptoms	Treatment	Prevention
Urinary tract infection	Infection of the bladder, kidneys, ureters, urethra. Causative or contributing factors: bladder distention and urine stasis, poor instrumentation technique, inadequate equipment cleaning, decreased hose resistance, alkaline urine, low fluid intake	1. Rising temp 2. Hematuria 3. Foul smelling urine 4. Dysuria 5. Turbidity 6. Low back/flank pain 7. Elevated spasticity 8. Anorexia, fatigue 9. Diaphoresis	1. Increase fluid intake 2. Indwelling catheter 3. Antibiotics	1. Proper technique and consistent schedule with urine bladder catheterization 2. Regulate fluid intake and cath schedule to avoid bladder distention 3. Urinary antiseptic and Vit. C to lower pH
Calculi	Calcium or other mineral deposits lodged in any portion of urinary tract. Precipitating factors: infection, immobility, urine stasis	1. Hematuria 2. Turbidity 3. Low back/flank pain 4. Increased spasticity 5. Diaphoresis 6. Often accompanied infection	1. Cystolithopaxy 2. Percutaneous lithotripsy 3. ESWL 4. May pass stone spontaneously	1. Increase mobility 2. Lower urine stasis and residual 3. Increase fluid intake

	infection, lower tract obstruction		irrigation and mechanical obstruction of catheter	3. Lower sphincter resistance with medication, sphincterotomy
Detrusor sphincter dysynergia	Hypotonic bladder and sphincter, simultaneous detrusor sphincter contraction. Associated factor: incomplete SCI	1. Difficulty voiding 2. Increased residuals 3. Reflex	1. Lioresal 2. Dibenzyline 3. Minipress 4. Anal sphincter stretch	——
Autonomic hyperreflexia	Exaggerated autonomic response to noxious stimulus below level of SCI. Occurs in SCI about T6	1. Headache 2. Hypertension 3. Bradycardia 4. Diaphoresis 5. Congestion & chills 6. Blurred vision 7. Flushing above lesion	1. Raise head of bed 2. Remove noxious stimulus, i.e., empty distended bladder 3. Anticholinergic medication 4. Peripheral dilating medication	1. Regulation and monitoring of intake and output 2. Proper positioning or urine equipment 3. Measures to prevent infection and calculi
Penile scrotal fistula/urethral diverticula	Fistula at penoscrotal junction or urethral diverticula caused by indwelling catheter irritation	1. Difficulty inserting catheter 2. Often accompanied by infection	1. Remove indwelling catheter 2. May require suprapubic cystotomy	1. When indwelling cath required insert smallest size possible 2. Tape cath to lower abdomen in male, upper thigh in female

9

GASTROINTESTINAL MANAGEMENT

PHYSIOLOGY OF DEFECATION

Defecation results from the action of the defecation reflex augmented by the sacral cord reflex. These reflexes can be inhibited or facilitated by voluntary control. With the defecation reflex, feces in the rectum distend the rectal wall. This initiates afferent impulses that spread through the myenteric plexus, initiating peristaltic waves in the descending colon and sigmoid, and forcing feces toward the anus. As the peristaltic wave approaches the anus, the internal anal sphincter relaxes. When the external sphincter is voluntarily relaxed, defecation occurs.

Because the defecation reflex is extremely weak, it is fortified by another reflex involving the sacral cord segments and the autonomic nervous system. Rectal distention stimulates the afferent fibers which transmit impulses to and from the sacral reflex center via the pelvic (parasympathetic) nerve. These impulses, traveling back to the rectum, greatly intensify the peristaltic waves, increase abdominal pressure, relax the internal sphincter, and make the defecation reflex more effective.

With the voluntary pathway, awareness of defecation occurs when increased peristalsis and internal sphincter relaxation stimulate the pudendal nerve, which sends impulses up the spinothalamic tract of the spinal cord to the brain. The brain then sends impulses back down the corticospinal tracts to initiate the valsalva maneuver, which increases intra-abdominal pressure, increases straightening and elongation of the colon, moves the feces into the rectum, and relaxes the internal and external sphincters. An alternative action from the voluntary pathway is inhibition of the defecation reflexes through inhibition of the external sphincter.

TABLE 9.1 Neurogenic Bowel Classification Related to SCI

Classification	Description	Pathophysiology
Reflex (spastic, hypertonic, automatic, upper motor neuron)	Impaired perianal sensation, impaired awareness of urge, intact bulbocavernosus reflex and sphincters, reflex incontinence	Neurological damage above sacral reflex center 2° to SCI
Areflexic (autonomous, lower motor neuron)	Diminished or absent perianal sensation, awareness of urge, internal sphincter intact, absent external sphincter response, absent bulbocavernosus reflex, incontinence 2° to flaccid external sphincter	Neurological damage to sacral reflex arc 2° to conus medullaris, cauda equina, or peripheral nerve injury, myelomeningocele, or tumor below S2–S4

Sympathetic stimulation (T6–L3) can also inhibit defecation by decreasing peristalsis and contracting the internal anal sphincter.

PATHOPHYSIOLOGY

Bowel function can be adversely affected by preexisting diseases such as diverticulitis, colitis, and Crohn's Disease. Bowel function can also be impaired as a result of disruption in the neurological control mechanisms secondary to brain lesions, spinal cord lesions, and peripheral nerve damage. Neurogenic bowel classification associated with SCI is reviewed in Table 9.1. Gastrointestinal complications are reviewed in Table 9.2.

IMPLEMENTING A BOWEL MANAGEMENT PROGRAM

A bowel program should be designed for each individual based on present elimination patterns, eating habits and preferences, activity level, lifestyle, support system, coping abilities, and the type of disability and how this has affected functional abilities, plus the goals that have been mutually defined and the potential level of patient cooperation. This information is then integrated into the

TABLE 9.2 Gastrointestinal Complications

Complication	Symptoms	Etiology
Constipation and impaction	Loss of appetite, nausea, diaphoresis, headache, abdominal discomfort/distention, decreased bowel sounds, infrequent, irregular evacuation pattern	Decreased mobility, muscle weakness, inadequate diet, decreased bowel tone, medications
Diarrhea	Loss of appetite, nausea, diaphoresis, abdominal cramping if sensation present, hyperactive bowel sounds, frequent watery stools	Dietary changes, antibiotics, virus
Autonomic hyper-reflexia	Subjective: headache, diaphoresis, chills, nasal congestion, chest pressure, nervousness Objective: hypertension, bradycardia, diaphoresis, flushed face	Bowel impaction, instrumentation, disimpaction
Paralytic ileus	Abdominal distention, absent bowel sounds	Occurs within 24–48 hrs. after SCI possible 2° to sudden cessation of autonomic innervation
Peptic ulceration and GI bleed	Hematemesis, guaiac positive stool, decreased hg, hct and BP, increased HR	May occur within 7–10 days after SCI 2° endogenous release of steroids, steroid administration, and increased HCl production from unopposed vagal stimulation

following basic components of a neurogenic bowel management program.

Diet

Implement the necessary diet and fluid intake modifications to insure that the individual is receiving an adequate amount of bulk, roughage, and fluid. Bulk is needed for the production of well-formed stools. Foods high in bulk include whole grain products such as bran, whole wheat, and cornmeal. Ingestion of large quantities of bulk foods without adequate fluid intake (approximately 2000 cc per day) for lubrication can create impaction problems. Stimulants will help intensify the peristaltic action of the bowel. Roughage in the form of fresh fruits and vegetables provides some of this stimulation as well as bulk. Particularly helpful for their stimulating effects are prunes, figs, and dates. Spicy foods, caffeine, and alcohol also provide an irritant type of stimulation. Foods that tend to constipate include such items as white rice, white potatoes, white pasta, cheese, and chocolate.

Timing

Establish a regular schedule of rectal stimulation and/or toileting. (Rectal stimulation increases colon peristalsis and produces a more complete emptying of the lower bowel. It may be contraindicated in patients with cardiac conditions.) When possible, take advantage of the gastrocolic reflex which occurs 15 to 30 min. after each meal. Use the same time frame as the individual's previous evacuation pattern if possible. In establishing an effective schedule, consideration must be given to the individual's lifestyle and the amount of assistance that may be needed.

Positioning

Facilitate evacuation by having the individual in a position that is anatomically conducive for elimination, either sitting with the knees higher than the hips or left sidelying. Augment weakened or paralyzed abdominal muscles by use of abdominal massage, an abdominal binder, and supporting the individual in a leaning over position. If some abdominal muscle strength is present and there are no cardiovascular contraindications, encourage the individual to use the abdominal muscles to bear down.

Activity

Encourage increased activity appropriate to the individual's tolerance and functional level to counteract the constipating effects of immobility. Work with the physical therapist and occupational therapist to facilitate maximum mobility and independence in bowel management activities.

Medications

If bowel results are inadequate and inconsistent in spite of implementing corrective dietary, scheduling, activity, and positioning measures, medications such as stool softeners, gentle stimulants, and bulk laxatives may be needed. (Note: Adequate fluid intake is required when using stool softeners and bulk laxatives.) Harsh laxatives and enemas should not be used on a regular basis as they can lead to long-term management problems.

Other medications can also have an effect on the function of a neurogenic bowel. For example, narcotics and antacids containing aluminum hydroxide can be constipating. Anticholinergic and sympathomimetic medications can also decrease GI motility. Antibiotics can decrease the normal GI flora which can result in diarrhea. It may be necessary to re-evaluate the medication regime if any of these medications are creating problems and determine if adjustments can be made to reduce or eliminate the bowel disrupting effects.

Managing and Preventing Complications

Paralytic ileus: Insert a nasogastric tube (NGT), connect it to low suction, and keep the patient NPO until bowel sounds return.

Peptic ulceration and GI bleed: In newly injured patients *guaiac* all stools, monitor vital signs, and evaluate bloodwork daily for any significant changes. Administer antacid and/or histamine H_2 antagonist as ordered by physician.

Constipation: Review fluid intake (increase as needed) and diet (increase fiber, decrease constipating foods). Assess need for medication changes (decrease anticholinergics, increase softeners and/or stimulants). Review schedule, activity, positioning, and stimulation techniques and make changes as needed.

Impaction/obstruction: Check bowel sounds. Palpate abdomen. Assist in obtaining an abdominal flat plate. Administer oral laxatives and enemas. With complete obstruction the patient may require temporary NGT insertion and gastric decompression to prevent vomiting and subsequent aspiration until the obstruction is eliminated.

Diarrhea: Review with the patient any dietary factors that may have caused or contributed to the problem. Encourage adjustments as needed and review the rationale with the patient. If diarrhea is related to antibiotic therapy, diet adjustments and the addition of unsweetened yogurt may be helpful. Provide scrupulous skin care after each bowel movement. If the diarrhea is severe, additional causes may need to be explored. Fluid and electrolyte replacements may also be needed.

Autonomic hyperreflexia: Assist the patient to a partial sitting position. Insert a local anesthetic cream into the rectum 10 minutes prior to disimpacting. Monitor vital signs frequently as the stimulation of the disimpaction process may further exacerbate the symptoms and raise the blood pressure. Oral laxatives may be needed to move a high impaction. Anticholinergic or vasodilating drugs may be necessary to reduce symptoms and ease the patient's discomfort. Assist the patient in learning the symptoms and causes of hyperreflexia and prevention measures such as maintaining a well regulated bowel routine.

The preceding guidelines are applicable to each type of neurogenic bowel. However, the management emphasis will vary slightly. For example, the person with a reflex bowel will be more responsive to the stimulation of a suppository or digital than will the person with an autonomous bowel. Those individual are likely to have more difficulty establishing a successful routine and need to put additional emphasis on diet and intra-abdominal maneuvers while maintaining a regular evacuation schedule. Scheduling remains a crucial factor for the person with an uninhibited bowel, but rather than focusing on stimulation of the reflex arc as with the reflex bowel, the focus is on stimulating conscious awareness and control of the reflex activity. A behavior modification approach may be beneficial in this situation.

SUMMARY

In the stage of acute care, the gastrointestinal management focuses on prevention of the secondary problems of a paralytic ileus or gastrointestinal bleed. Thereafter, the emphasis shifts to regaining bowel "control" through a predictable routine. Aberrations in one's routine can be extremely frustrating and humiliating experiences. Assist the person with spinal cord injury in learning his body's responses to the many variables that contribute to a successful routine, and encourage him to adhere to those proven guidelines. Restoration of predictability or "control" will help to reestablish his self-confidence.

10

SKIN CARE

ANATOMY AND PHYSIOLOGY

Skin, the body's largest organ, is composed of a sequence of layers, which together provide for its varied features. The outermost layers offer protection from the elements. The subsequent layers allow for secretion, excretion, insulation, sensation, and thermoregulation. Hair and nails are considered "accessory organs."

Protection

As long as the skin is intact, it provides a barrier that protects the individual from foreign organisms or toxins. Problems arise when there is a disruption in the protective barrier, such as trauma or infection.

Secretion, Excretion, and Thermoregulation

Sweat glands and sebaceous glands eliminate toxins, lubricate the skin, and regulate body temperature. The sebaceous glands emit an oily substance that protects the skin and helps it retain moisture. These secretions decrease with age, so an older person usually has dry skin. Young people, on the other hand, tend to have oily skin from hyperactive glands. Sweat secretions dissipate heat as well as remove toxins. The hairs and tiny muscles that surround them assist in thermoregulation. Subcutaneous tissue, which connects the skin with underlying muscle, provides insulation, thus conserving body heat.

Sensation

There are four different cutaneous sensations: hot, cold, pain, and pressure. The differences of sensation are achieved through different receptors located throughout the body. For example, there are concentrations of specialized nerve endings in the fingertips that respond to temperature changes by sending impulses to the brain via afferent fibers. The cortex then interprets and integrates the messages and sends a motor response via the efferent fibers. There also are reflex responses which act on the cutaneous information alone and furnish an immediate response. Sensation is achieved through both the specialized cutaneous receptors and interpretation of the cortex.

EFFECTS OF SPINAL CORD INJURY AND PREVENTION GUIDELINES

Risk Assessment

Any patient with impaired abilities is at risk for developing a pressure ulcer. Using a validated risk assessment tool, evaluate the patient and develop a corresponding treatment plan. Risk factors include compromised physical and/or mental condition, impaired sensory perception, decreased mobility, incontinence, moisture, compromised nutrition, friction and shear. Reassess the patient at routine intervals to ensure treatment is appropriate.

Loss of Mobility

Spinal cord injury and the resultant immobility provide many threats to the integrity of the skin, both directly and indirectly. Directly, the skin is subjected to prolonged pressure, friction, heat, and moisture. Indirectly, it is compromised by nutritional deficits, chemistry imbalances, and renal and cardiovascular complications.

To minimize these threats a good prevention program is essential. Initially, after the method of spinal column immobilization has been assured, establish a schedule of position changes. Periodically reassess this turning schedule to accommodate any changes in the patient's tolerance. Make schedule revisions in 30-min. increments and closely monitor the skin response.

When positioning a patient in bed avoid pressure to bony areas if possible. Evaluate for the type of protective equipment appropriate for the individual. For example, someone who is well nourished with good skin integrity may need only a sheepskin, whereas an undernourished person with sensitive skin may need a water mattress and other protective devices.

When he is sitting in a wheelchair, a patient needs frequent position changes. Leaning forward, shifting from side to side, and pushing up are beneficial, providing one or both ischials are free of pressure for at least 30 s during each maneuver. When the individual is not able to shift his weight independently, he will need a wheelchair cushion providing as much pressure relief as possible, plus the assistance of another person. Wheelchairs with a motorized recline enable the patient with high quadriplegia to change position independently.

Loss of Sensation

Sensory deficits may vary in type and degree. For example, some patients experience a loss of temperature sensation but can identify deep and light pressure. Others may experience a total loss of sensation. Because of these sensory deficits, examine the skin thoroughly at least once a day, giving particular attention to bony prominences such as the ischial tuberosities, sacrum, coccyx, greater trochanters, ankles, heels, and elbows. As soon as possible the patient should assume this examination responsibility so that he learns his own skin tolerance. If unable to perform an independent examination with a long-handled mirror, he can instruct others to assist him.

Additional precautions may be necessary, based on the type of sensory deficit. Inability to interpret temperature can result in serious burns. Potential hazards include hot water, heaters, water pipes, cigarettes, and the sun. Proprioception allows the person to know where his body is in relation to space. With a disruption in this feedback, the spinal cord injured person may be unaware, for instance, that his foot is off the footrest. Any such situation can be hazardous initially until the person is able to compensate by using other discernible clues.

Impaired Circulation

Compromised circulation can result in peripheral edema and poor oxygenation, with subsequent tissue damage (see Chapter 6). Provide the patient with elastic support stockings and periodically elevate his legs to help alleviate or reduce this edema. Advise him to avoid wearing tight shoes and clothing. Care must be taken to prevent additional trauma to fragile edematous tissue during transfers and positioning.

Diaphoresis

As stated previously, the sweat secretions serve to remove toxins, assist in thermoregulation, and lubricate and moisten the skin. SCI patients do not sweat below the level of their lesion in response to an elevated environmental temperature; however, they may sweat profusely due to other medical complications. Because of this, keep the skin clean and dry to avoid maceration, which enhances bacterial growth.

Nutrition

In addition to the previous guidelines, nutrition plays a key role in preventing skin problems. Provide the patient with a high-protein diet (100 grams daily) that includes vitamin- and mineral-rich fruits, vegetables, and grains (see Chapter 7).

Equipment

To provide additional skin protection, select the proper type of wheelchair seating system and bed covering. These devices are assistive in nature and do not substitute for position changes. Ideally, they should mold to the individual's contours or provide flotation to equalize pressure distribution. They should allow for the passage of water vapor so moisture does not stay on the skin. They should be financially and practically suited for the individual's lifestyle, as well as being durable and comfortable. Proper maintenance is essential for any protective equipment used. Skin problems can be caused if flotation devices are under- or overfilled, if foam or gel devices become deformed, if foam becomes wet, if gel becomes overheated, and if improper coverings are used on any of the cushions.

Special beds also are available to provide skin protection through regular rotations. These include the Stryker Wedge® and

Roto-Rest® discussed in Chapter 6. The Clinitron® air-fluidized bed is designed especially for skin care. It consists of a system in which air is pumped through a bed of tiny glass beads. A special covering supports the patient over this cloud of circulating air and beads. The Kinnair® bed is another air fluidized system designed for patients at high risk for skin breakdown or for pre or postop surgical repair of pressure ulcers. The Kinnair® bed is fully motorized for ease of patient care; the mattress consists of air chambers covered with a gortex-like fabric. The air chambers distribute air to accommodate the patient's body contour, thus reducing capillary pressure over bony prominences.

In addition to seating systems, bed coverings, and special beds, there are a variety of devices available to protect particular parts of the body, such as elbows, heels, and ankles. The needs of the individual patient determine the selection of all equipment.

PRESSURE ULCER MANAGEMENT

A pressure ulcer can result from any one or a combination of etiologies: pressure, heat, moisture, and friction. Generally, a red area or other indications of tissue deterioration such as swelling and heat herald the formation of any ulcer. The manifestations evolve from damage to the capillary supply to that tissue. If the discoloration does not fade within a reasonable amount of time (15 to 30 min.), take precautions to avoid further pressure to the area. First, determine the source of the problem. If the source is pressure, then remove the pressure from the area. Then determine the extent of damage to the tissue and choose a treatment. After a particular treatment has been initiated, allow reasonable evaluation time before changing to another type of treatment, unless there is an immediate adverse reaction evident. In addition, take measures to protect any open decubitus from contamination.

Concurrently, carefully evaluate the patient's nutritional status. Any draining wound is losing protein at a time when the body's protein requirements have increased in an attempt to heal the wound. If blood tests indicate a negative nitrogen balance (see Chapter 7), protein supplements may be necessary along with a high-protein and vitamin-enriched diet.

The care of a pressure ulcer cannot be an isolated activity.

Carefully review causative factors, since patterns of behavior and routines may need redirection to prevent the skin problems from becoming chronic.

The wound will pass through stages of healing. The capillaries dilate to provide more circulation and nutrition to the wound. Leukocytes are attracted to the area to evacuate the dead cells. A fibrin web is formed around the edges and is filled in by fibrocytes from surrounding subcutaneous tissue. As the edges slowly begin to fill in, the epidermis is stimulated to grow. If contaminants and necrotic tissue are interfering with this healing process, debridement may be necessary. This may be accomplished either by surgical or chemical means. Also check for tracts or signs that the area is healing over, leaving open canals underneath. If necessary, use loose packing to prevent this problem from occurring and to promote healing from the inside out.

After the inflammatory response has halted and the capillary surge has subsided, collagen is laid down to form scar tissue. As the collagen ages, the bonds become firmer and the scar acquires tensile strength; however, this tissue may not be as hearty as the original tissue and should be checked frequently.

Methods of Treatment

There are numerous treatments for pressure sores. A brief overview is included here. Check your institution's protocol and vendor instructions before making decisions.

Stage I is a nonblanching erythema of intact skin. This is the "heralding sign" for pressure ulcers. Treatment includes:

A. Refer to the risk assessment and plan; implement aggressive preventive measures.

B. Apply transparent or hydrocolloid dressings to protect area and prevent further tissue injury.

Stage II is a partial thickness skin loss involving the epidermis:

A. Re-assess preventive measures.

B. Cleanse wound with normal saline.

C. Apply transparent dressing to blistered areas or wounds with minimal exudate. Follow product instructions carefully and evaluate patient's response to the product. Document using objective measurements.

D. Apply hydrocolloid or calcium alginate dressings to wounds with moderate exudate. Follow product instructions, evaluate and document as above.

Stage III is a full thickness wound with damage to subcutaneous tissue and perhaps underlying fascia:

A. Remove any necrotic areas through the following means:

1. Surgical debridement.

2. Chemical debridement: Cleanse wound with normal saline. Soften or incise eschar, then apply prescribed enzyme treatment. Cover with a dry dressing. Repeat 2–3 times daily until the wound is clean.

3. Mechanical debridement: Cleanse wound with normal saline. Apply a wet to damp gauze dressing. Repeat three times daily until wound is clean.

4. Physiologic debridement: Cleanse wound and cover with transparent, hydrocolloid, or calcium alginate dressing according to manufacturer's instructions.

B. For clean wounds with moderate drainage:

1. Cleanse wound with normal saline.

2. Apply hydrocolloid or calcium alginate dressings according to manufacturer's instructions.

3. For heavy exudate, apply wet to damp dressing as above.

Stage IV is a full thickness wound with damage to muscle, bone, or supporting structures:

a. Obtain surgical and nutrition consultations.
b. Evaluate for infection and treat accordingly.
c. Treat wound as for Stage III treatment.

Cleansing Agents.   Normal saline provides a gentle irrigation of the wound without counteracting other treatments.

Antiseptic, Antibacterial Agents.   Some protocols call for the use of povidone iodine, peroxide, dakins solution and others to cleanse wounds of bacteria. Use caution with these agents as they may have harmful effects on wound healing. The use of these agents should be prescribed by a physician who has current knowledge regarding pressure ulcer treatment.

Moisturizers and Emollients.   Apply these agents conservatively to restore the skin's moisture level and do not massage bony prominences.

Topical Circulatory Stimulants.   These products are intended to improve circulation to the wound and therefore promote wound healing. As with all products the wound should be reassessed frequently and progress documented in an objective manner.

Semipermeable Dressings.   These topical dressings allow oxygen to the wound while providing for moist wound healing. Many of these dressings are also transparent and allow visualization of the wound. Apply these dressings carefully avoiding any wrinkles which may cause further tissue damage. Redress the wound every three days, when the periphery seal is broken, or the area has been soiled.

Hydrocolloid Dressings.   These are occlusive dressings for moist wound healing. Most agents "melt" into the wound, absorbing wound drainage and providing gentle debridement as the dressing is removed.

Calcium Alginate.   These dressings are based on a composition and facilitate wound healing. They are applied as the hydrocolloid and transparent dressings.

Drainage Absorptive Agents.   Most of these products are designed to work with the calcium alginate and hydrocolloid dressings to absorb more exudate and penetrate deep wounds.

SUMMARY

Although skin care may not take priority with the newly injured patient, the prevention of decubiti is a lifelong concern. This area of personal care, once managed automatically, now requires conscious planning to compensate for the alterations in mobility and sensation. However, instruction and experience will facilitate the integration of these care requirements into the patient's daily activities. Additional surveillance will be required to accommodate the changes associated with aging: nutritional, circulatory, endocrine and postural compromises.

11

MUSCULOSKELETAL
CONSIDERATIONS

Following a spinal cord injury, an individual will have lost partial or total muscle power below the level of the lesion. As a result of this paralysis or paresis, he may not be able to perform many of the independent activities that he previously took for granted, such as walking and feeding, grooming, and dressing himself. Regaining independence in the performance of these and a multitude of other activities are the primary goals of both the person with SCI and the health professionals who work with him. His ability to achieve these goals depends on a number of factors: the innervated musculature and the strength of those muscles are revealed in a manual muscle test, whether he has any limitations in range of motion, whether spasticity is present, the size and proportion of his body, and the emotional investment he has in the goal or task.

This chapter will present an overview of the levels of muscle innervation, complicating factors that may influence functional capabilities, guidelines for preventing these complications and for performing transfers and a review of technological advances. The reader is referred to physical and occupational therapy textbooks for in-depth discussions of therapy programs and equipment.

SPINAL LEVELS AND
FUNCTIONAL POTENTIALS

Tables 11.1 and 11.2 describe the potential muscle function and skills possible for different levels of SCI. The muscle groups mentioned are the most important for that level, although some muscles may be innervated at more than one level. These descriptions

TABLE 11.1 Spinal Cord Segments and Corresponding Muscles/Movement

Spinal Cord Segment	Muscle(s)	Movement
C1–3	neck muscles	limited head control
C4	diaphragm	diaphragmatic breathing
	trapezius	shoulder shrug
C5	deltoid	shoulder abduction
	partial biceps	partial elbow flexion
C6	extensor carpi radialis	wrist extension
	biceps	elbow flexion
C7	triceps	elbow extension
	extensor digitorum	finger extension
C8	flexor digitorum	finger flexion
T1	hand intrinsics	finger abduction, adduction
T2–T12	intercostals	deeper inhalation
T6–T12	abdominals	forceful exhalation
		increased trunk stability
L1–L2	iliopsoas	hip flexion
L2–L3	hip adductors	hip adduction
L3–L4	quadriceps femoris	knee extension
L4–L5	tibialis anterior	ankle extension
L5	extensor hallucis longus	great toe extension
S1	gastrocnemius/soleus	plantar flexion
	hamstrings	knee flexion
S1–S2	flexor digitorum	toe flexion
S2–S4	bladder, lower bowel	elimination

are presented only as general guidelines. As indicated previously, there are many other emotional and physical factors that will influence each person's functional capabilities.

SPASTICITY

Spasticity is one of the factors that can influence a patient's functional ability. Although the pathophysiology is not fully understood, evidence suggests that it is partly due to increased central excitability of the isolated spinal cord below the injury, following the release of inhibitory impulses from the brain. It is character-

TABLE 11.2 Neurological Levels and Functional Potential

Level	Activity
C1–4	Dependent in feeding, grooming, dressing, bathing, bowel and bladder routines, bed mobility, transfers, and transportation. Independent wheelchair propulsion with pneumatic or chin control and with electronically adapted communication and environmental control devices.
C1–3	Dependent on ventilation support.
C5	Independent feeding and grooming with adapted equipment. Dependent in dressing, bathing, bowel and bladder routines, and transportation. Requires assistance for bed mobility and transfers. Independent wheelchair propulsion in motorized chair and with electronically adapted communication and environmental control devices.
C6	Independent feeding, grooming, upper extremity dressing, bathing, bowel routine, and bed mobility—all with adapted equipment. Requires assistance for lower extremity dressing and bladder routine. Potentially independent transfers with transfer board. Independent manual wheelchair propulsion with plastic rims or lugs indoors. Independent driving with adapted van. Independent phone operation and page turning with equipment.
C7	Independent feeding, grooming and bathing with equipment. Potentially independent in upper and lower extremity dressing and bowel and bladder routines. Independent bed mobility, transfers with or without board, manual wheelchair propulsion, driving with adapted car or van and in communication activities.
C8–T1	Independent in all personal care activities, bed mobility, transfers, wheelchair propulsion, driving with adapted car or van, and in communication activities.
T2–T10	Independent in all activities. Ambulation with long leg braces and crutches or walker for exercise only (nonfunctional).
T11–L2	Independent in all activities. Potentially independent functional ambulation indoors with long leg braces and crutches.
L2–S3	Independent in all activities. Independent ambulation indoors and outdoors with short leg braces and crutches or canes.

ized by alterations in neuromuscular performance, such as increased muscle tone, heightened stretch reflexes, and exaggerated flexor muscle movements following a noxious stimulus.

Spasticity usually begins to appear about six weeks after a cervical injury and 10 weeks after a thoracic injury, reaching a plateau within one to two years. Almost all patients with cervical injuries will have spasms, and the majority of those with thoracic injuries will have some degree of spasticity. Less than half of the patients with lumbar injuries and less than a fourth of those with cauda equina injuries will have spasms. Many individuals with incomplete injuries tend to have more severe spasticity than those with complete injuries. This involuntary action may override any remaining voluntary motion.

Though generally considered to be a nuisance, some spasticity can be of benefit to the individual by maintaining muscle tone, facilitating transfers, and triggering voiding. A variation from one's "normal" degree of spasticity would signal other problems creating increased stimulation, such as a bladder infection or a decubitus.

Ongoing health problems and poor positioning can result in severe debilitating spasticity. This condition then will result in further complications; for example, strong flexor spasms can lead to the development of contractures, making daily care and positioning difficult; while a strong extensor spasm can eject a person from a bed or chair, causing serious injury.

In cases like this, methods may be explored to reduce or alleviate the spasms. Unfortunately, no agent or technique has been found to be totally successful. The responses to spasmolytic agents such as diazepam (Valium), dantrolene sodium (Dantrium), and baclophen (Lioresal) vary considerably. Implanted intrathecal baclophen delivery systems have been tried experimentally in selected centers throughout the country. Preliminary results have been encouraging, and a wider distribution has been approved. The benefits of decreased spasticity must always be weighted against the potentially harmful side effects of the medications.

If preventive health care measures, medication management, and physiotherapy techniques (proprioceptive neuromuscular facilitation, reflex inhibition patterning, splinting, icing, heat) prove unsuccessful, it may be necessary to do motor point blocking. In this procedure a 6% phenol solution is injected into a motor point of a given muscle causing lysis.

If motor point blocks are unsuccessful, surgical procedures such as a neurectomy (interruption of peripheral nerve), longitudinal myelotomy (division of connections between anterior and posterior horns), rhizotomy (division of anterior and posterior spinal nerve roots) may be performed.

SKELETAL SYSTEM CHANGES

Changes in the skeletal system can lead to various medical complications. Some of these changes also can affect a patient's functional ability.

Bone mass (calcium and phosphorous) is constantly being dissolved and replaced. Much of the stimulus for this process comes from the stress of weight-bearing activities. Following an SCI this weight-bearing ability is usually lost. Serum calcium and phosphorous levels rise and an increased amount of calcium is spilled into the urine, leading to the development of urinary tract calculi. Bone mass continues to decrease, leading to osteoporosis and a greater potential for fractures.

Heterotopic ossification is another condition resulting from the change in bone-regenerating activities. Calcium lost from the bones is deposited in skeletal muscle and tendons (myositis ossificans) or around joints (periarticular ossification). Signs that one of these conditions may be developing include swelling and heat in a particular area, pain if sensation is intact, and increasing limitations in range of motion of that particular extremity. Views on treatment vary from limiting movement to providing active therapy to the involved area. Some individuals may benefit from the medication Didronel®, which limits the formation of the calcium deposits. Others may need surgery to remove the mass after the formation process has plateaued, as indicated by X-ray comparisons and alkaline phosphatase levels.

To prevent or minimize any of the complications occurring from skeletal changes, provide the patient with an active therapy program, weight-bearing activities on a tilt table or similar device, and guidance on overall health maintenance.

RANGE-OF-MOTION EXERCISES

As stated previously, functional capabilities can be altered by diminished range of motion (ROM), which is the degree of movement at each joint. Movement restrictions can result from either bony changes or from tightness of the muscles or supportive tissues around the joint. Daily ROM exercises, either at bedside or in the therapy department, are important preventive measures. The motions described here are for one direction of movement. Return to the original position by reversing the directions.

Shoulder Movements

Refer to Figure 11.1a and c while reading these instructions.

1. Flexion/extension
   a. Hold the patient's forearm with one hand; with the other hand, grasp the top of his shoulder joint to stabilize it.
   b. Move his arm from the side of his body up and over his head, with the palm of his hand facing the body and his elbow relatively straight.
2. Abduction and adduction
   a. With one hand holding his elbow joint, support his forearm; with the other hand, stabilize his shoulder joint.
   b. Move his arm away from his body along the surface of the bed.
3. Internal and external rotation
   a. Hold his forearm with one hand; with the other hand, stabilize his shoulder.
   b. Roll his forearm down toward the bed surface in front, then back (upper arm is twisting the shoulder joint).

Elbow Motions

Refer to Figure 11.1b

1. Flexion/Extension
   a. Hold his upper arm with one hand and his forearm with the other.

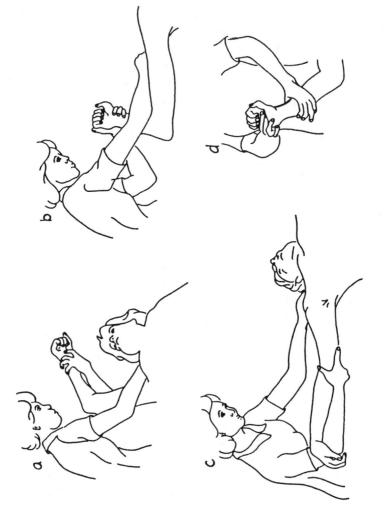

Figure 11.1 Range-of-motion exercises of the upper extremities: (a) shoulder motions, (b) elbow extension, (c) shoulder adduction, and (d) wrist flexion.

    b. Bend his elbow joint to bring his forearm up toward his upper arm.

  2. Supination/Pronation
    a. Use the same hand position.
    b. Twist his forearm until his palm faces up, then twist until his palm faces down.

Wrist and Hand Motions

Refer to Figure 11.1d

  1. Extension/flexion
    a. Hold his forearm with one hand; place the thumb and fingers of the other hand on opposite sides of his palm.
    b. Bend his wrist back to about 90° (fingers will straighten naturally).

Hand ROM varies depending on the level of remaining muscle function. In general, if no muscles are active at the wrist then the fingers can be stretched open to lie flat. However, if wrist muscles are present, the fingers should not be stretched. They should be allowed to curl naturally, since this will give the hand added function (tenodesis).

Back Stretching

If spasticity or tightness is present in the back muscles, stretching may be necessary. If there is no tightness, do not perform this exercise, as it may cause overstretching. Figure 11.2 illustrates this maneuver, which is a simple matter of positioning the patient sitting with his legs straight in front and then gently pushing him forward until his arms reach beyond his feet.

Hip Movements

As the legs are heavier than the arms and somewhat harder to manage, it is easier to use a combination of arms and body when doing ROM with the hips. Refer here to Figure 11.3.

  1. Flexion
    a. With one arm, cradle his leg with the knee bent; with the other hand grasp his hip joint for stabilization.
    b. Lift his leg up toward his chest. Do not allow his hip to

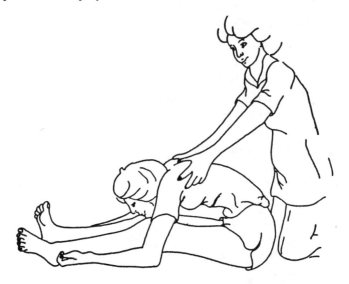

Figure 11.2   Back stretching in the long-sitting position.

twist during this movement; his foot should stay in a straight line with his hip and not swing in or out.

    c. For straight-leg stretching, support his leg on your shoulder with one hand. Holding his knee with the other hand, stabilize his hip joint. Raise his leg straight up to approximately 90°.

2. Abduction/adduction
    a. With one arm, cradle his straight leg with your hand holding his knee; with the other hand, stabilize his hip joint.
    b. Move his leg along the surface of the bed away from the other leg to approximately 45°.

3. Internal/external rotation
    a. Place one hand on his thigh and the other hand below the knee.
    b. Roll his leg inward until his kneecap faces the other leg; then roll his leg outward in the opposite direction. (Leg stays straight in alignment and rolls like a log.)

Knee Motions

While doing ROM of the hip, the knee also will receive ROM (see Figure 11.3). Unless specifically instructed, this is sufficient. The

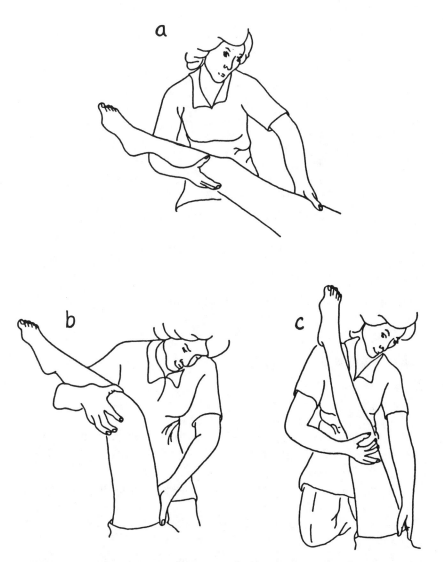

Figure 11.3 Range-of-motion exercises of the lower extremities: (a) abduction of the hip, (b) flexion of the hip and knee, and (c) straight-leg stretching.

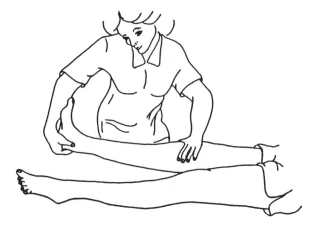

Figure 11.4   Heel-cord stretching.

knee should be free to bend for a total range of approximately 90–120°.

Ankle Motions

Refer to Figure 11.4

1. Heel-cord stretching.
   a. Place one hand on his knee to prevent it from bending; the other hand cradles his heel, with the sole of his foot resting on your forearm.
   b. Push the sole of his foot forward, stretching the muscles in the back of the leg. The heel cord can be very difficult to stretch, and you may need to lean your body weight forward to help stretch it.
2. Other ankle motions: To exercise all other ankle muscles, grasp his foot and move it in a circle (up, in, down, out).

ORTHOTIC DEVICES

In addition to the range-of-motion exercises, orthotic devices can provide protection from debilitating contractures and can maximize the functional abilities of the patient with weak hand and

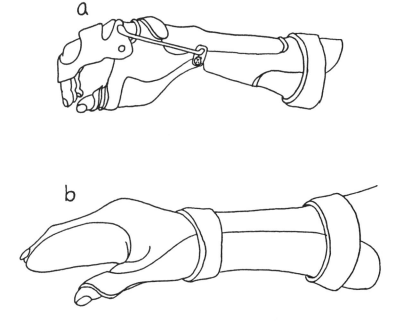

Figure 11.5 Orthotic devices: (a) tenodesis splint and (b) resting splint.

wrist muscles. These devices may be prefabricated or made by the individual institution. Most of them are simple and versatile, as the following examples illustrate.

1. If the patient's shoulders and arms are weak, they may need support when he is sitting in the wheelchair initially. A lapboard of wood or Lexon® plastic can be fitted to the chair arms to provide such support. The lapboard also affords a table surface for activities when table heights are too low or too high to be useful.

2. If his wrists are weak, a resting splint or an ADL (Activities of Daily Living) leather wrist support will protect and support his muscles (see Figures 11.5 and 11.6). If hand and finger functions are compromised, the following universal components can provide additional assistance for performing light self-help activities like feeding, grooming, and writing. See Figure 11.7 for illustrations.

   a. The ADL orthosis has a C-clip swivel and utensil

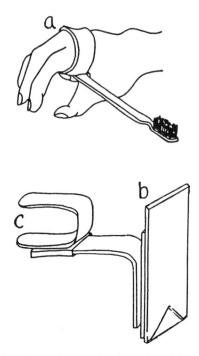

Figure 11.6   Devices for activities of daily living: (a) a universal cuff, (b) vertical holder, and (c) C-clip.

pocket. This device will support the wrist, substitute for grasp, and provide stability to a variety of implements such as a spoon, fork, and toothbrush.

b. The universal ADL cuff has a pocket to hold standard implements. An elastic strap holds it securely around the hand, thus providing a simple holding device.

c. The universal C-clip swivel ADL cuff is a basic holding device, easily put on with a swivel pocket for utensils. Functional wrist motion is necessary for its use.

d. The universal vertical holder provides an ADL pocket attached to an L-shaped strip of metal. When used with the previous three devices, it positions eating and writing implements in a vertical (rather than horizontal) position.

e. The universal folding extension handle with ADL cuff compensates for elbow and forearm motions by provid-

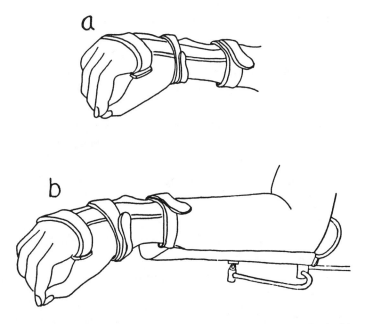

Figure 11.7   Dorsal wrist splint (a) and balanced forearm orthosis (b).

ing reach and positioning. It can be inserted into the ADL pockets of any of the other devices.

TRANSFERS

The method a patient uses to move to and from his wheelchair will be influenced by the same factors that affect his other functional capabilities: the muscles that are innervated and their strength, the degree of spasticity, any ROM restrictions that exist, his body size and proportion, and his motivation.

All transfers described here are ones in which the patient needs full assistance. It usually is easier for two people to lift someone from a wheelchair; however, this is not always practical and there are various ways that one person can perform a transfer easily.

Good body mechanics are a most important part of transfer activities. This minimizes the chance of straining muscles while lifting and provides for a smoother, safe transfer. Always consider these points:

1. Keep your knees bent and back straight. Never lift with your knees straight, as this puts too much strain on your back.
2. Keep your feet apart with one leg as close as possible to the person being lifted and the other placed in the direction you are moving.
3. When two people are doing the transfer, the stronger person should lift from behind the wheelchair.
4. Coordinate the efforts with one person giving directions.
5. Always properly align and prepare the wheelchair and the patient before beginning a transfer.
6. Be sure the wheelchair is locked!

Two-Person Transfer

Refer to Figure 11.8.
   Preparation.

1. Move the chair parallel to the bed and as close as possible. Lock the wheelchair.
2. Remove the adjacent armrest and the swing-away foot pedals.
3. Lifter #1 holds the patient under his arms and grasps above his wrists. This both controls balance and provides a hold for lifting. (Alternative method is grasping the sides of his pants belt with him leaning back against lifter's arms.) Lifter #2 positions one arm under the patient's legs as close as possible to his buttocks and places the other arm under his lower legs.

   Lift.

1. Have your legs in the proper position. The top person can place one leg on the bed for better positioning.
2. Lift together by partially straightening knees to a semi-standing position and shifting weight toward bed.

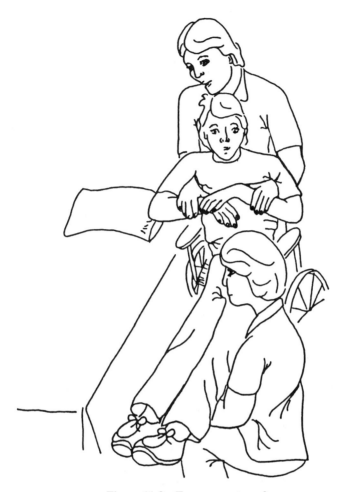

Figure 11.8   Two-person transfer.

3. Lower the patient to the bed surface by bending knees. Do not bend forward at the back.

One-Person Transfer, without Sliding Board

Refer to Figure 11.9.
Preparation.

1. Position the wheelchair at a 45° angle to bed. Lock the wheelchair.

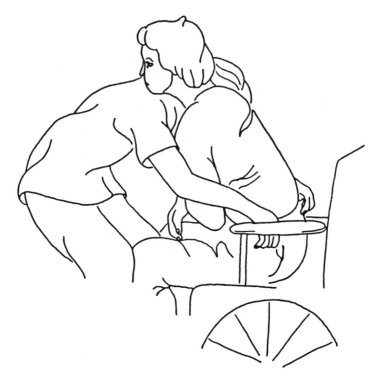

Figure 11.9   One-person transfer without sliding board.

2. Remove the adjacent armrest and the swing-away foot
   pedals.
3. Slide the patient forward in the wheelchair until his buttocks are forward from the wheels.

Lift.

1. Lean the patient forward so his chin rests on your shoulder. The patient's arms should be folded in his lap or hug-
   ging your neck, is possible.
2. Grasp the back of his pants or belt and squeeze his knees
   with your knees. Always keep your knees bent.
3. To lift, rock back on bent knees, bringing the patient's
   weight forward over his feet. In one swift motion, lift and
   pivot him toward the bed, keeping your knees bent.

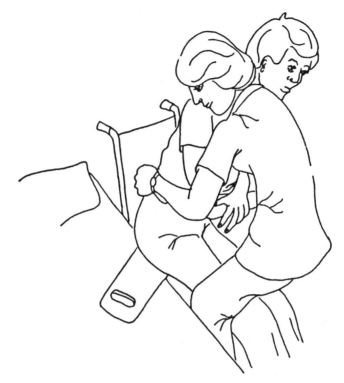

Figure 11.10   One-person transfer with sliding board.

4. Lower the patient to the bed by bending your knees further.

One-Person Transfer, with Sliding Board

Refer to Figure 11.10
Preparation.

1. Position the wheelchair as for the previous transfer.
2. Twist the patient in the wheelchair so his buttocks are closer to the bed and his knees point away.
3. Place the sliding board, half under his buttocks and half under his thigh, being careful not to dig the board into his skin. Angle the board toward the end of the bed to form a bridge.

Transfer.

1. Use the same arm and leg position as in the previous transfer.
2. Rock back on bent knees, leaning the patient's weight forward over his feet. His buttocks should remain in contact with the board, as this is a sliding transfer, not a lift.
3. Slide the patient along the board as you pivot toward the bed. This can be done in one continuous motion or in several small movements, whichever is more controllable.

One-Person Transfer, Hoyer Lift®

Refer to Figure 11.11.

1. Roll the patient onto one side and place the sling on the bed. The sling extends from his shoulders to his thighs. Roll him back on top of the sling.
2. Attach the hooks to the sling.
3. Pump the lift up until his buttocks clear the bed surface. He will be in a sitting position. Adjust the sling if necessary for better sitting posture.
4. Roll the lift to the wheelchair so that the legs of the lift can pass on the outside of the large wheels.
5. Center him over the wheelchair seat and lower him slowly. As he descends, his knees may need to be pushed backward so that his hips are to the rear of the chair seat.

TECHNOLOGICAL ADVANCES

Functional electrical stimulation (FES) is one of the latest developments in musculoskeletal management. It consists of electrical stimulation to certain muscles with a biofeedback component. The process is controlled by computers. The purpose of FES is to improve muscle strength and/or to prevent atrophy, to improve functional abilities, to control spasticity, and to increase cardiovascular endurance. Ambulation is the most publicized area of FES success. These ambulation systems frequently combine the FES unit with reciprocating gait orthoses and a walker. However,

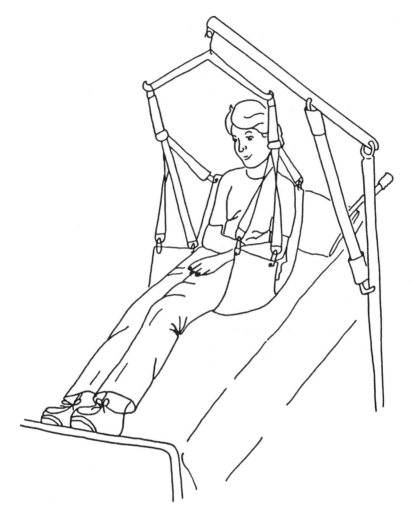

Figure 11.11   Hoyer Lift® transfer.

they are only available at selected research centers at this time. Other FES equipment is becoming more available in regional SCI centers and for home use in the forms of the Regys and Ergys ergometers. Ergometers are computerized bikes that send a sequence of electric currents to paralyzed muscles in the lower extremities. This stimulates them to move the bike pedals against resistance. Until recently, individuals with incomplete injuries and with injuries below T10 were not eligible candidates for FES. Now a device called the neurosignal amplifier provides some of the benefits of FES without the discomfort.

Other technological advances have significantly increased independence for persons with quadriplegia. These include power wheelchairs, computers, environmental control systems, robotic workstations, and home automation systems. Depending on the device, control options include pneumatic, voice, eyeblink, and microswitch operation.

SUMMARY

Any loss of mobility can limit a person's ability to perform many self-care tasks that we generally take for granted, such as grooming, eating, and moving from place to place. To relinquish one's independence is often a dehumanizing experience. By preventing further limitations and supplying him with appropriate devices, staff members can assist the patient in minimizing his dependence and concurrently will reinforce his self-esteem.

12

PSYCHOLOGICAL AND EDUCATIONAL CONSIDERATIONS

INTRODUCTION

After a SCI a person experiences a multitude of losses which lead to major disruptions in the physical, psychological, and social dimensions of his life. In addition, his ability to use previous problem solving, self care, and coping skills may be severely compromised and his goals and personal relationships abruptly altered. These changes are likely to result in a variety of feelings including fear, anger, resentment, confusion, helplessness, and inadequacy.

Adjusting to SCI is a highly individualized, dynamic, evolving process reflecting the person's ongoing effort to restore and maintain physical, psychological and social integration and balance, and to positively redefine himself and his life within the new context. Family members also experience lifestyle disruptions and an evolving process of adjustment.

This chapter will provide an overview of factors affecting the adjustment process and the related facilitation techniques. Because a major part of this process involves ongoing education, the variables influencing learning and teaching will also be discussed.

FACTORS AFFECTING ADJUSTMENT

For rehabilitation professionals to be able to enhance a person's coping abilities and facilitate the adjustment process they must be sensitive to the multitude of factors that influence each individual. The following list highlights some of the factors to be considered:

- Demographic information including age, marital status, occupation, education level, ability to read and write, primary language, and financial status.
- Cognitive information including brain disease or injury related impairments (attention deficits, memory deficits, impaired abstraction, generalization, concept formation, and problem solving abilities, language disturbances, and executive deficits); learning style, level of intelligence, history of learning disability, perceived information needs and priorities, current level of knowledge about disability, health expectations, and past experiences that may prepare for present learning.
- Physical information including musculoskeletal limitations, diminished visual and hearing acuity, reduced tolerance secondary to pain, fatigue, and/or deconditioning.
- Psychological information including presence of affective disorders related to brain damage, presence of fear, anxiety, and depression; type and effectiveness of coping style; level of maturity; self image; personal meaning of disability; response to previous health care experiences; history of alcohol or drug abuse; outlook on life; locus of control.
- Sociocultural information including support systems; age, health, and availability of significant others and their roles; family dynamics; religious influences; cultural background; social and ethnic values; attitudes and beliefs of family and peers and their reactions to patient's disability; living arrangement; lifestyle; possible conflicts between culture and therapeutic recommendations.

Factors that may compromise the adjustment process include poor physical health, chronic fatigue and pain, external locus of control, poor self esteem, lack of a support system, and limited coping skills.

Factors aiding adjustment include emotional maturity, flexibility in coping patterns, good self esteem, family support, job and financial security, and being less physically inclined. Young people have the advantage of adaptability but are likely to have the disadvantage of emotional immaturity and self identity confusion.

THE ADJUSTMENT PROCESS

Patient Reactions

During the initial period following a SCI the individual is confronted with an overwhelming set of circumstances. He has experienced a sudden dramatic change in almost every aspect of his life. Feelings of helplessness and fear are exacerbated by a multitude of unknowns in his immediate environment. Pain, fatigue, isolation and medications can further compromise his overburdened coping abilities. In an effort to manage the unbearable stress, he may temporarily regress or attempt to restructure and regain control of his environment through various behavioral methods, such as resistance to medical and therapeutic recommendations. Emotional stability, self doubt, approach avoidance behavior, regression, and denial may also be manifested during this stage. In the past denial and regression were considered maladaptive responses. In most circumstances they are now viewed as functional coping mechanisms that can help the person from being overwhelmed and allow him time to regroup psychologically.

Many of the emotional reactions demonstrated during the acute phase will continue into the rehabilitation phase though the life and death issues are usually less prominent. Over time a degree of emotional stability is restored.

In the past, psychological literature has been dominated by the stage theory that compares reactions of persons facing new disabilities with those facing death. In recent years the literature has challenged the stage theory by emphasizing the tremendous variability in response to SCI. However, a general understanding of adjustment variables can enhance the rehabilitation professional's sensitivity to some of the underlying issues the patient is facing and the possible behavioral manifestations. A person may vacillate between feelings of helplessness and panic, to detachment and controlled constructive thinking. In his efforts to adapt he may search for meaning in what has happened to him and attempt to regain mastery over his life.

Some studies have concluded that persons who manifest less depressive affect during rehabilitation had more successful outcomes. Other studies also support the concept that the absence of depression soon after injury onset does not prognosticate a poor adjustment to the disability (Trieschmann, 1988). In fact, true clinical depressions occur in only a small percentage of patients, though most experience a grief response.

Family Reactions

The family members of a person with SCI also experience severe emotional disruptions as a result of the injury. Finding the reality too painful and overwhelming to accept, they may temporarily deny the permanency of the disability and its consequences. Initially, there may be doubts whether their injured relative will even survive. Fear and anxiety may make future planning impossible at this point.

Frustration at not being able to help improve the situation may be manifested as angry criticism of the staff. The family's continuing fear and anxiety may elicit either overprotective behavior toward their relative, or isolation from him.

As the implications of a permanent disability become more evident, many different responses may be seen. Some families begin seeking desperately for cures. Others maintain a false cheerfulness when with their injured relative to avoid burdening him with their sadness and anxiety. They also may avoid talking about their outside activities so that he will not be reminded of his losses. They may feel angry at him for this disruption to their lives, a feeling that often will elicit feelings of guilt, which further increase their overall anxiety and emotional discomfort. Role changes, economic worries, and physical exhaustion contribute further stresses to the overburdened family.

Facilitating the Adjustment Process

To implement a plan to facilitate psychosocial adjustment:

- Provide decision making opportunities that foster autonomy and self confidence.
- Provide guided practice in problem solving to help promote self confidence. Often hospital environments tend to suppress problem solving and decision making opportunities.
- Provide experiential and group discussion opportunities to

assist in dealing with role changes and altered social relationships, in order to decrease feelings of isolation and hopelessness, and to enhance communication skills.
- Simplify tasks when appropriate so the patient will be successful and will receive positive reinforcement. Success at physical and psychological tasks can blend into success at social reconditioning.

The following are examples related to these suggestions:

- Encourage the patient to participate in the planning of his schedule and in prioritizing learning activities.
- Offer open-ended questions on diet, fluid intake, scheduling, activity, and medications to help the patient identify the cause and remedy of a bowel management problem.
- Role playing within a group and recreational activities outside of the rehabilitation setting are helpful experiential opportunities.
- Tasks such as dressing can be simplified by selecting clothing that is easy to put on, such as sweatsuits or apparel that has been adapted to the individual's abilities.
- Help the patient identify psychological and cognitive strengths while deemphasizing the focus on physical limitations.
- Throughout the rehabilitation process, continue to assist the patient in identifying and acquiring new self concept definers.

EDUCATIONAL CONSIDERATIONS

The overall rehabilitation plan needs to provide the learning opportunities and supportive atmosphere to increase the patient and family's knowledge and understanding of the physical and psychosocial effects of SCI, and to enhance their coping skills.

The foundation of such a plan is incorporated in a multidimensional education program (see Appendix III - Patient Family Teaching Overview). This program must address the physical, cognitive, psychological, and sociocultural dimensions of their lives and offer opportunities for them to learn new skills and adaptive behaviors. Because of the tremendous variations in neurological status, abilities, and life circumstances, teaching plans must be individualized to meet the unique needs of each person.

The rehabilitation professional has an integral role in all aspects of patient and family education. Primary responsibilities within the role include facilitating learning through the use of appropriate teaching and rehabilitation methodologies and providing a caring environment that is supportive of each individual's personal exploration and growth.

Definitions of Learning and Teaching

Learning is the acquisition of knowledge, attitudes, and skills that lead to behavioral changes. It is a dynamic, multidimensional process influenced by a person's previous life experiences and current psychological and physical status. Learning is motivated by the individual's attempt to resolve unmet problems or needs.

Teaching is the plan of action that is designed to bring about learning or that allows it to occur. The process of teaching has the same basic components as the nursing process. An assessment is made of the patient's and family's learning needs, motivation, and ability to learn. Following the assessment, learning objectives are established. A teaching plan is then developed based on the assessment data and learning objectives. After implementation of the teaching plan, its effectiveness is determined by evaluating whether the adaptive behaviors have been achieved.

Factors Affecting Motivation and Ability to Learn

Many factors affect a person's motivation and ability to learn. These include neurological status, developmental level, and locus of control. A person with SCI who has also sustained a traumatic brain injury will have a variety of cognitive deficits affecting learning potential depending on the areas and extent of brain damage. The motor and sensory deficits associated with SCI can interfere with psychomotor learning and affect the type of teaching methods used. Pain can adversely affect the individual's motivation and ability to concentrate and attend to learning activities.

The adolescent learner tends to be egocentric and self absorbed. Striving for peer approval, privacy, and independence are major developmental concerns. After sustaining a disability, the ability to resolve these concerns may be seriously compromised. The young and middle aged adult learner desires immediacy of application of teaching; needs to integrate new ideas into established patterns; may have some limited knowledge of learning materials but this may be distorted by misconceptions; is reality and problem oriented, and is concerned about preserving self-esteem. With the aged learner, maintaining independence is a prime learning motivator. Imprinting new learning requires more time and the use of association and previous learning. Sensory impairments may interfere with learning. Information tends to be processed better visually rather than auditorially. Other characteristics include physical limitations (in addition to disability-related limitations) of decreased strength, endurance, and speed; impaired perceptual ability with decreased vision and hearing; and egocentricity with well-established patterns.

A person with an internal locus of control tends to feel in control of life's events, copes better with threatening situations, and perceives the relationship between behavior and the results. He tends to be focused on long-term gains and is more willing to forego immediate rewards to achieve these. He usually responds well to health promotion and independent study programs. A person with an external locus of control tends to feel helpless and powerless in the face of problems. These feelings of helplessness and powerlessness are further reinforced after the individual has sustained a disability. He usually responds best to structured group programs.

In addition to neurological status, developmental level, and locus of control, the individual's level of fatigue, anxiety, depression, fear, denial, and anger can all affect his motivation and ability to learn. Conflicts associated with health and cultural beliefs and values, interpersonal influences, time constraints, financial problems, and the complexity of the management plan can also adversely affect a person's motivation and ability to learn.

Planning and Implementation

To develop an effective patient and family education program the rehabilitation professional must obtain pertinent information regarding the learner's demographic, cognitive, physical, psychological, and sociocultural status. The planning and implementation process should then become an integration of this information, the identified learning needs, and the appropriate subject content and teaching methodologies.

- With the patient and/or family establish realistic learning goals and objectives and measurable time-related outcomes. Goal achievement is more likely when these goals are related to the self-identified needs of the learner. Also realistic, attainable goals provide mechanisms for feedback, which motivates further learning.
- If conditions such as pain, fatigue, or anxiety interfere with the individual's learning readiness, work with him to reduce or eliminate the problem by implementing or modifying pain management techniques, by modifying rest and activity schedule, and by providing stress management instruction and counseling. If cognitive deficits limit the individual's ability to learn, include the family or other care givers in all teaching interventions.
- Select the subject content that fulfills the learning objectives and is appropriate to the learner's cognitive, physical, and psychological capabilities. Determine the number of sessions required by breaking the content down into meaningful parts.
- Prioritize information of practice based on the immediacy of the learning needs. The need is acute if the individual will be in physical or emotional danger without the information or response. Preventive needs apply to information or responses that are needed to eliminate or decrease the possibility of illness or complications. Maintenance needs relate to self-care information and activities.
- Organize the content presentation or practice from simple to complex. Organize information from concrete to abstract. Begin with what the learner knows and build on this.
- Select teaching strategies appropriate to the learner's learning style, locus of control, developmental level, and gender (discussion/lecture, verbal presentation/demonstration, group/individual instruction/independent study).

- Pace learning activities according to the learner's physical tolerance and cognitive abilities.
- Select instructional materials to supplement the teaching methodology based on the learner's cognitive, visual, and hearing abilities, learning style, verbal/reading comprehension. Provide opportunities for follow-up discussion when audiovisual or printed materials are used.
- Provide repetition until the learner demonstrates mastery through correct return demonstrations and/or verbal feedback.
- Provide family members of the cognitively impaired patient with information to help them understand the nature of the problem and the pathophysiological reasons for the patient's behavior. Assist them in learning how to work with the patient to maximize abilities, minimize disability-related limitations, and prevent complications. (see Zejdlik (1992) and Hanak (1986, 1992) for further information on traumatic brain injury management and family teaching.)
- Provide a physically comfortable learning environment that is temperature controlled, well lit, easily accessible, and free of visual and auditory distractions.
- Convey attitudes that will enhance learning: value the material being taught, convey interest in teaching, and demonstrate acceptance of the learner.
- Provide ongoing feedback to facilitate learning, promote self confidence, and further motivate the learner.

Evaluation

Evaluating learning involves comparing the expected learning outcomes with the learner's actual behavior following teaching. Evaluations are also used to judge the effectiveness of the teaching and the appropriateness of the teaching materials.

When giving feedback to the learner during or following the evaluation, the rehabilitation professional should initially provide positive reinforcement for the desired behavior before discussing areas that still need improvement. Absolutes like "always" and "never" should be avoided. When information is shared, alternatives should be presented so the learner can make some independent decisions. When specific suggestions are offered, the rationale for each should be given. Feedback should be given as soon as possible after the evaluation. When providing feedback to the patient with brain damage use feedback mechanisms that he is most responsive to in light of the specific cognitive impairments. An example would be providing tokens that could then be redeemed by the patient for a desired special activity.

In addition to the evaluation of the learner, the teaching program and the professional's role must also be evaluated to facilitate future program planning and presentations. The following questions address this broader evaluation dimension:

- Were the goals mutually agreed upon, realistic, and timely?
- Were educational needs adequately identified and defined?
- Were the results of the learner assessment taken into consideration when developing the teaching plan?
- Was the learner's self respect and sense of control maintained?
- Was positive feedback given on an ongoing basis?

Staff Reactions

Working with persons with SCI elicits a wide range of emotional responses in staff members. They are required to have technical expertise, skill in communication and interpersonal relations, knowledge of resources, an understanding of the multiple psychological ramifications of the disability, and the ability to integrate these dimensions into a sensitive, individualized plan of care. To many, the rewards of this type of work are deep and unquestionable, but this does not negate the fact that the emotional burdens are tremendous and can take a toll on the most dedicated health professional.

We first must take a look at our own reactions and methods of coping before we can provide effective guidance and support for the patients. Too often our anxieties, sadness, and hopes may interfere with our ability to accurately assess the patient's status and needs. Working with a person who has suffered a massive assault on his body integrity can elicit an identification response. Fears surface of the possibility that this could happen to us, that we may be as vulnerable as he is. The emotional fragmentation that many injured individuals demonstrate can arouse further fears of our own emotional stability and how our self-concept could be shattered like theirs.

The stress of these unspoken or unidentified fears may elicit a complex series of defense mechanisms. To protect and isolate ourselves from the fears, moralization and intellectualization may be used.

Feelings of anxiety and depression are common when one is confronted with the dependency and other losses suffered by the patient. In efforts to relieve our own emotional discomfort we may send conflicting messages to him. On one hand, he is expected to conform to the hospital regime and be docile and dependent. Rule breakers or those individuals who try to direct their own programs are termed uncooperative. At this same time, in our own eagerness for improvement, we may be pushing him to be independent and responsible before he is ready. He may need the time to be sad and to be protected and taken care of. We also may unconsciously present disincentives by withdrawing attention from an individual as his independent skills increase and by redirecting our focus to the one who needs us more.

Nurses and therapists, because of the close and frequent contact with the person with SCI, may frequently be the object of displaced feelings such as anger. Threats, insults or obscene gestures may be the only way for the patient to vent his feelings. It is imperative that we remain professional and not react on a personal level. Ensure the patient's safety and leave the room. Ask a colleague to cover for you until you regain composure. Indicate to the patient that this is not acceptable behavior and offer the opportunity to rechannel his feelings through participation in diversionary activities and/or a counseling program. Continuity of caregivers is essential in making positive, forward gains for this patient. A token system or contract may enable the professional to praise positive behavior and learning and discourage antisocial behavior. Team coordination for such systems is also essential. Frustration and loss of esteem are other emotional hazards that we may encounter if we are not able to help the patient meet his goals or our own. This can create increased tension with patients, families, and co-workers.

Since most of us have entered helping professions because we want to make people better, these feelings of inadequacy and personal failure can have effects reaching far beyond the immediate situation. Our motivations also can have long-lasting effects on the patient—in our desire to be needed and helpful we may be sending a message subconsciously that discourages his efforts to gain independence.

SUMMARY

The preceding sections of this chapter have discussed possible psychological responses of patients and their families to SCI and psychosocial and educational interventions to facilitate the adjustment process. It must be emphasized that the generalizations are simply tools to assist us—the primary focus of our efforts remains with the individuals and how they feel about themselves.

To provide patients and their families with the most effective, consistent, and sensitive support, the health care team must formulate a plan that takes into consideration all the multiple dimensions and circumstances of their lives. These include socioeconomic and cultural background, support systems, educational level, preinjury occupation, past experiences with illness, past coping skills, present level of stress, and the effectiveness of present coping behavior.

As indicated previously, our own emotions can seriously compromise our abilities to provide optimum care. Therefore, it is essential that we periodically reassess our motivations and responses to determine their therapeutic effectiveness. Also, by this periodic reevaluation and self-exploration we may tap resources in ourselves that will give an even greater depth, warmth, and sensitivity to all of our interactions—and in such an atmosphere the patients and their families may find the strength and acceptance they need to successfully adjust to the multiple changes in their lives.

13

SEXUAL CONSIDERATIONS

Sexuality is a complex concept—an integration of an individual's body image, beliefs, goals, attitudes, relationship to others, and the physiological components of his or her sexual activities. Sexual roles and behavior are further influenced by the person's age, sex, and sociocultural environment. Sustaining a disability can dramatically affect a person's sexuality as it often forces a reexamination of all these aspects of self. For example, many people with disabilities develop a poor self-image as they may feel self-conscious about their physical limitations and unable to fulfil previously defined roles and goals. These feelings can lead to or worsen the depression and anger they may already be feeling at what has happened to them. Interconnected with the poor self-image and depression is often the fear of rejection. The person's negative behavior in anticipation of rejection can result in this fear becoming a reality. Fear of a bowel or bladder accident can further reinforce poor self-image and fear of rejection. Another fear is that sexual activity will cause pain or precipitate medical complications. Guilt about overburdening a partner with extra responsibilities can also affect an intimate relationship.

The able-bodied partner may be experiencing similar feelings—depression and anger over role and lifestyle changes, fear that sexual activity may injure the partner, and guilt over changed feelings toward the partner and over feelings of anger and resentment. Fatigue is another major factor for the able-bodied partner, who may have assumed many additional responsibilities.

Because of these and other physical and psychological issues, the individual with a disability and his/her partner will need a variety of supportive interventions from the rehabilitation nurse and other members of the rehabilitation team to help them achieve a satisfying sexual readjustment. These interventions include offering individual and couple counseling and educational opportuni-

[handwritten margin notes: poor self image, physical limitations, depression, anger, rejection, negative behaviour, impotent, guilt]

ties and facilitating peer group discussions. To provide effective sexual counseling and education, the nurse and other team members must have an understanding of their own sexuality including their sexual values, biases, and problem areas; sensitivity and concern for the patient's and partner's feelings and needs; the ability to listen; and a knowledge of how the psychological and physiological aspects of sexuality are affected by the disability.

SEXUAL RESPONSE CYCLE

Masters and Johnson have divided the sexual response cycle into four phases for both males and females: excitement, plateau, orgasm, and resolution. Stimulation is needed to begin the excitement phase. This stimulation can come from almost any source, with the mind being the primary one. Touch (particularly in the sensitive erogenous zones) and vision both play lesser but still important roles. Other senses such as taste and smell have varying degrees of importance for each individual.

With continued stimulation the plateau phase may be reached. Here sexual tensions are intensified and orgasm may be experienced. During orgasm the build-up of muscle tension and vascular engorgement are released. After this release, the resolution phase begins and the individual returns to a relaxed, unstimulated state.

Two key differences in the male and female are that the female can often achieve multiple orgasms and her sexual responses usually involve more of her body. For males sexual pleasure is usually more centered in the penis. Also, males experience a refractory period after orgasm, during which further stimulation will not lead to another orgasm.

The frequency and type of sexual intercourse are determined by the couple's preference and to some extent by societal influences. Respect and sensitivity for each person's feelings are fundamental aspects of any sexual counseling role.

SEXUAL PHYSIOLOGY IN THE MALE
WITH A SPINAL CORD INJURY

The man usually experiences significant changes in his sexual physiology following a SCI. Depending on the level and severity of the injury, erection and ejaculatory ability and fertility may be compromised. Sensory deficits also may affect his ability to achieve orgasm.

Erection and Ejaculation

The ability to get an erection and ejaculate are controlled by nerves that originate in the lowest part of the spinal cord (segments T_{12} to L_2 and sacral levels 2, 3, and 4).

Psychogenic erections (see Figure 13.1) result when messages are passed down the spinal cord from the brain to the sacral area. The brain sends out these messages because of stimuli received through the senses of sight, sound, and smell, as well as through the imagination and memory. If the spinal cord is injured someplace between the brain and the area controlling sexual response, the messages usually will stop just before the lesion and the man thus affected will be unable to achieve a psychogenic erection. However, men with a lower-level or incomplete lesion are able to obtain this type of erection. This is possible because the message from the brain may bypass the injured portion of the cord via the autonomic nervous system in the sacral region.

Reflexogenic erections (see Figure 13.2) result from direct stimulation of the genital area. They are called reflexogenic because they are controlled by a reflex arc between the genital area and the cord via the pudendal nerve (see Chapter 1). Since this arc does not need messages from the brain in order to function, it can continue to operate in the portion of the cord below the injury.

Spontaneous erections occur when some internal stimuli initiate the reflex. For instance, a full bladder may be sufficient to cause an erection. However, since the individual cannot control when they will occur, these types of erections are not as important in sexual activity as the reflexogenic or psychogenic variety.

Ejaculation, which is a motor function, cannot take place if the particular nerves and parts of the spinal cord controlling it are injured. Few cord injured men are able to ejaculate spontaneously.

When looking at the presence or absence of these elements of male sexual function, some generalizations can be made. The first is that the level of injury can influence sexual function. Usually, erection is elicited more commonly in men with high levels of spi-

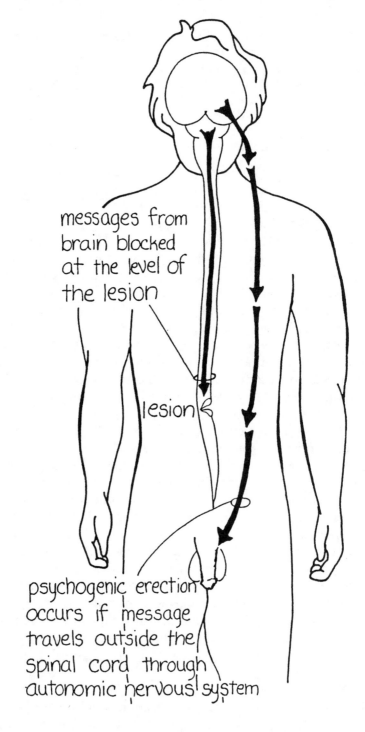

messages from
brain blocked
at the level of
the lesion

lesion

psychogenic erection
occurs if message
travels outside the
spinal cord through
autonomic nervous system

Figure 13.1   Neurophysiology of psychogenic erections.

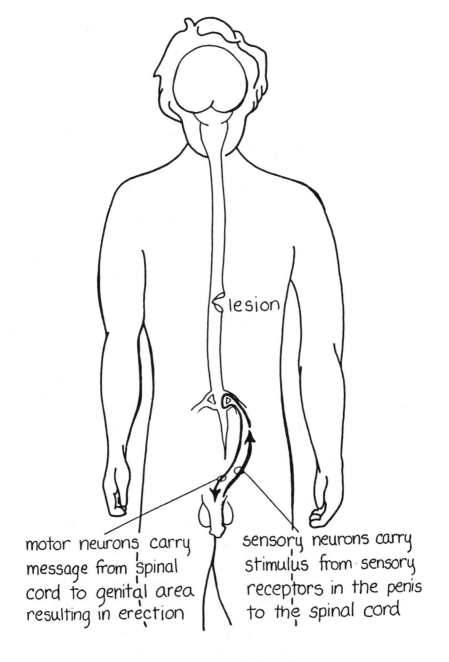

lesion

motor neurons carry
message from spinal
cord to genital area
resulting in erection

sensory neurons carry
stimulus from sensory
receptors in the penis
to the spinal cord

Figure 13.2   Neurophysiology of reflex erections.

nal injury. Conversely, ejaculation is present more commonly in those with lower-level injuries and may occur in the absence of erection. Secondly, genital sexual function also can be influenced by the extent or completeness of the lesion; men with incomplete lesions have greater preservation of all aspects of their genital function. However, partial damage may interfere with reflex activity and may permit inhibiting influences of the brain to interfere with reflex responses. Thirdly, some elements of sexual function are more vulnerable than others; orgasm and ejaculation are much more vulnerable than erection itself. Therefore, there can be greater differences between a paraplegic and a quadriplegic, in the types of genital sexual function remaining, especially in those with incomplete lesions.

It is important to note that, depending upon the level of injury, the stimuli that produce an erection may differ. Men injured high in the spinal cord usually have reflex erectile response to tactile stimulation, whereas those injured in the lower part of the cord may be able to respond only to stimulating thoughts (if the T_{12-12} segments are still intact).

Orgasm

The incidence of "classical orgasm" seems to occur in a very small percentage of men with spinal cord injuries. When it does occur, the incidence appears to parallel that of emission and ejaculation. However, many men describe experiences which, while not like orgasms they experienced prior to injury, are nonetheless very pleasurable and are defined by them as the high point of a particular sexual experience.

Management Options for Erectile and Ejaculatory Dysfunction

For the man who is experiencing erectile dysfunction as a result of his disability, penile prostheses are available. The three main types include the semirigid silicone rods, which give a permanent semi-erect penis, flexible silicone rods which can be bent into position for intercourse, and the inflatable prosthesis, which can be maximally inflated to achieve a full erection when desired. Psychological counseling and a complete physical assessment are required to determine if the man is an appropriate candidate for a prosthesis and, if so, to determine which type would most effectively meet his needs.

Another option for managing erectile dysfunction is with the use of vacuum tumescence such as the Erecaid System. This system is composed of a plastic cylinder, tubing, a vacuum hand pump, and rubber constriction/retention bands. A vacuum is produced in the cylinder which then draws blood into the corpora of the penis, producing engorgement and rigidity. A structured patient education program and adequate practice are necessary before the device is issued.

For the man with erection and/or ejaculatory dysfunction there are three methods under investigation for achieving erection and for triggering ejaculation for sperm evaluation and artificial insemination. These methods include electrical stimulation, chemical stimulation with injections of papaverine, phentolamine, or prostaglandin E-1 in the spongy erectile tissue of the penis, and vibrator stimulation. At this time no consistently successful method has been discovered. For triggering ejaculation however, vibromassage appears to be the safest and most readily available method.

SEXUAL PHYSIOLOGY IN THE FEMALE WITH A SPINAL CORD INJURY

Research done on sexual physiology post SCI has focused primarily on men rather than women, partly because there are fewer females with SCI. Other reasons may be that the injury has less effect on a woman's physical ability to have intercourse and her fertility is not affected adversely.

Sexual Response

Since the endocrine glands are not under direct neurological control, women with SCI usually do not experience dramatically altered hormonal levels, and ovulation and menstruation continue on the same preinjury schedule. If a woman does miss some menstrual periods after her accident, she usually will resume her preinjury schedule within about 6 months.

Vaginal lubrication will vary depending on the level of the lesion. If the reflex is intact the reflexogenic function still should be there, but the psychogenic aspect would be lost. With lower motor neuron (LMN) lesions, reflexogenic lubrication would not be possible but psychogenic lubrication would be. Clitoral and vaginal response seem to follow a similar pattern—reflexogenic or psychogenic, depending on the level and completeness of the lesion.

Few studies have been done on genital sensory loss and the effects of female orgasm. One type of experience that some women have described is the phantom orgasm—a vivid imagery in dreams, even though they lacked genital sensation and subjective feelings of gratification. Other spinal cord injured women describe heightened arousal and orgasmic feelings from breast stimulation or from stimulation of other erotic areas above the level of the lesion.

Birth Control. Because fertility is not affected in many women with SCI, methods of birth control need to be reviewed. The birth control pill is probably the most widely discussed and debated method of birth control among members of the medical community. Except for sterilization it is the most effective method and is easy to use. However, studies reveal that pills with a high estrogen content cause a significant increase in the risk of blood clots in the able-bodied population. Unfortunately, no studies of the clot risk factor have been conducted with disabled women, but it is likely increased, as most of these women are already facing an increased clotting risk secondary to immobility. Other side effects to consider with progesterone/based birth control pills are weight gain and the depression some women experience, which may be magnified for the disabled women going through major lifestyle adjustments.

Another controversial, effective method of birth control is the intrauterine device (IUD). One potential complication of this method is pelvic inflammatory disease (PID). Pelvic pain and cramping are warning signs that this condition may be developing. The woman with SCI lacking abdominal sensation needs to be especially alert for other warning signs, such as spotting, temperature elevation, vaginal discharge, and possibly an increase in spasticity. Also, because women with IUDs often experience heavier menstrual periods, the woman on anticoagulant therapy should be aware of the potential complication of excess bleeding.

The safest methods of nonpermanent birth control are the diaphragm, sponge, and a condom-foam combination. While the diaphragm and sponge are relatively safe and effective, they do require manual dexterity to insert it properly. The rhythm method is preferred by some couples; however, this is usually less effective than the other methods and if a pregnancy is a definite health hazard for the woman, this would be an inadvisable choice.

Sterilization is a permanent method of birth control chosen by some women. Besides the psychological preparation needed, consideration must be given for the sterilization procedure with the least amount of physical stress.

Pregnancy

The woman with SCI who does not want children should seek out an obstetrician familiar with SCI. While her pregnancy will be similar to that of a woman without a cord injury, she still will need some special considerations.

A woman's body undergoes many physiological and anatomical changes to accommodate a growing fetus. Because of these changes and the resultant systemic strain, any woman with severe preexisting medical problems usually is advised to avoid pregnancy. Even a healthy woman is apt to encounter various problems resulting from her body's changing status. These problems include anemia, phlebitis, edema, blood pressure changes, urinary tract infections, constipation and impaired mobility. A prenatal program that includes a highly nutritious diet, daily rest periods, moderate exercise, positioning that facilitates venous return, and avoidance of hazardous medications can help prevent these problems and also protect the unborn child.

As previous chapters have indicated, a person with SCI is susceptible to many of the same problems that a pregnant woman may encounter. The preventive management guidelines are also similar. While the pregnant woman with SCI has an apparent double chance of developing any of these complications, she usually has the advantage of being more educated about her own body.

A unique consideration for the woman with SCI lacking abdominal sensation is that she may not be aware of when labor begins. Therefore, it is advisable that an earlier hospital admission be scheduled during the final weeks of her pregnancy to monitor the course of her cervical dilation. Since her contractions are hormone-controlled rather than neurologically controlled, paralysis will not interfere with them. However, forceps are often needed for deliveries since the woman lacking muscle power is unable to bear down during the final stages of labor and delivery. (As with any woman, pelvic anatomy usually determines whether a delivery will be vaginal or via Caesarean section.)

Another very important consideration is the danger of autonomic hyperreflexia (dysreflexia) occurring in the pregnant female with a lesion above T_6, especially during labor (see Chapter 4). An obstetrician unfamiliar with this phenomenon may make the mistake of associating an elevated blood pressure with a preeclampsia condition. As a rule, the woman experiencing dysreflexia symptoms during labor will have a blood pressure that fluctuates with each contraction, reaching a maximum at the time of delivery, then falling rapidly. Frequent blood pressure monitoring is essential to determine if this fluctuating pattern is present, as management will differ for each condition. If the hypertension of an autonomic condition reaches dangerously high levels during the contractions, spinal anesthesia should be administered.

SPECIAL CONSIDERATIONS

As discussed previously, the person with SCI does have some special considerations affecting the expression of his or her sexuality. Some involve the logistical problems that arise from sensory and motor changes, pain, spasticity, and bowel and bladder incontinence. To decrease the effects of these problems, more preparation is needed. This additional preparation and the resultant loss of spontaneity can become a problem itself, as one or both partners may feel that sex is just another chore.

For the person with compromised genital sensation, other techniques need to be explored to enable him or her to achieve sexual arousal and release. The primary methods involve using various forms of sensory amplification. To do this a person maximizes responsiveness to all the sensory avenues that are intact. This usually includes visual, auditory, and olfactory stimulation, as well as tactile stimulation of any sensory intact areas of the body. These physical stimuli, accompanied by sexual fantasies and other psychological stimuli, can increase the individual's level of sexual excitement to the point of orgasm. Those people who do not reach orgasm may still experience some of the physiological changes associated with the orgasm and resolution phases of the sexual response cycle. For the person with brain damage, the techniques to achieve sexual arousal will depend on the type and extent of his/her cognitive and behavioral deficits.

Communication. Open communication between partners is an essential element of all aspects of sexual interaction. Each partner needs to share what pleases and what does not in a physical sense. Equally important is the sharing and communicating of feelings of love, affection, and commitment.

Timing and Environment. As with any couple the timing of sexual activities and the environmental cues can greatly enhance or detract from the experiences. Since fatigue is a major factor for many people with disabilities and for their partners, an optimum time must be selected when both individuals are rested and not rushed. Also, for those individuals who have problems with spasticity, an optimum time may be when the spasms are reduced, such as after a warm shower or after receiving antispasticity medication. The optimum environment provides quiet, privacy, and other forms of sensory input that are sexually stimulating for the couple.

Personal Care. Because appearance has a major effect on how people view themselves and how others view them, patients should be instructed on how to most effectively manage hygiene and grooming tasks is relation to their disability-related limitations. Another consideration that may pose a problem is when the nondisabled partner is helping the disabled individual with his or her bowel and bladder routines. It may be difficult for him/her to have sexual feelings toward that person. It may be better in these cases for a visiting nurse or aide to handle such matters.

Positioning. Finding a position that will be comfortable, limit spasticity, and compensate for lack of mobility can be difficult. Many couples prefer a face to face sidelying position, as this allows them multiple sources of stimulation without placing either partner in a strained or dependent position. Some disabled individuals may achieve more functional movement by taking advantage of spasms. Others may experience more limitations because of them. Each couple needs to explore and find what is pleasing and acceptable to them. A waterbed is preferred by many, as it is more comfortable than a standard mattress and may maximize mobility for the partner with a disability.

Bowel and Bladder.   If a woman has an indwelling catheter, it is often easiest to leave it in but taped to the abdomen so it will not be pulled out. A man with a catheter can fold it back over the erect penis or allow enough slack for erection. A condom can then be applied. Women and men without catheters may prefer to limit fluid intake and to empty the bladder prior to intercourse. The possibility of a bowel accident occurring during sexual activity is a major concern for many persons with disabilities. Pre-planning is the best insurance to avoid having intercourse near the bowel routine time or when the routine has been greatly disrupted.

AIDS and Venereal Disease Prevention.   Preventing these diseases is a national concern for all population groups that are sexually active. Education on causes, symptoms, and preventive measures is applicable to both the able-bodied and disabled community.

SUMMARY

As stressed from the beginning of this book, respecting the individuality of each patient and being sensitive to his/her emotional needs are essential components of any aspect of SCI management. This is particularly evident in the area of sexuality, where the injured individual may have focused many of his/her doubts of self-worth and fears of the future. By encouraging verbalization of these feelings and providing information, encouragement, and positive reinforcement, staff members can create the atmosphere of concern and support that will enable each patient to rediscover his/her self-confidence and the promise of a fulfilling future.

GLOSSARY

abduction movement of segment of body away from midline

adduction movement of segment of body toward midline

adrenergic adrenalin producing

afferent nerves that carry sensory impulses to central nervous system

areflexic without reflexes

autonomic hyperreflexia exaggerated sympathetic response to noxious stimulus below level of lesion

axon part of neuron that conducts impulses away from cell body

Babinski sign reflex indicative of neurological pathology

bactiuria presence of bacteria in the urine

balanced forearm orthosis a wheelchair device that, by supporting the forearm, eliminates the force of gravity, thus enabling the person with limited arm musculature to perform such tasks as feeding and typing

belief systems classification based on how an individual receives, interprets, and integrates internal and external stimuli

calculi accumulation of mineral salts

cholinergic acetylcholine producing

Cloward procedure anterior cervical fusion

complete injury total paralysis and loss of sensation below level of injury

computerized axial tomography (CAT Scan) a noninvasive procedure that provides a more precise visualization of vertebral fractures and dislocations then standard X-rays

concussion impact injury resulting in partial or complete loss of function

contracture limiting joint deformity usually resulting from disuse and improper positioning

contralateral opposite side

contusion an injury to any part of the body where the skin remains intact

conus medullaris lower end of spinal cord

coping process whereby an individual under stress attempts to regain emotional equilibrium and freedom from stress-inducing disruption

cystogram a radiographic test of the bladder after the administration of dye

cystoscopy test performed by the urologist to examine the bladder with lighted instrument

cystourethrogram a radiographic test of the bladder and urethra, using an injection of dye

decubitus skin lesion usually resulting from prolonged pressure over a bony prominence

dendrite part of neuron that conducts impulses to cell body

detrusor the smooth muscle of the bladder

dyssynergia sustained or intermittent sphincter contraction simultaneously with detrusor contraction causing urinary retention

Doppler an ultrasonic flow detector used to diagnose phlebitis by determining whether a change in blood flow occurs during respiration (negative result)

dorsal wrist splint a leather splint that immobilizes the wrist in neutral alignment preventing overstretching of tendons

efferent nerves that carry motor impulses from the central nervous system to muscles or glands

environmental control unit (ECU) voice- or breath-activated unit that performs a variety of functional tasks

erythema a reddened area on the skin surface

F.E.S. (functional electrical stimulation) computer-organized electrical stimulation to paralyzed muscles

fiber tract bundles of axons having the same origin, termination, and function

fibrinolytic drugs medications that dissolve blood clots

flaccid absence of muscle contractions

fractional inspired oxygen (Fi_{O_2}) percentage of oxygen delivered to respiratory tract

fusion surgical procedure that stabilizes two or more vertebrae by constructing bone grafts between them

ganglia tissue containing groups of nerve-cell bodies located outside of brain and spinal cord

glossopharyngeal breathing method of breathing, using the mouth and throat, that forces air into the lungs

gray matter tissue composed of nerve-cell bodies; found in brain, spinal cord, and ganglia

Harrington rods metal distraction rods attached to vertebral bodies to aid in maintaining alignment

heterotopic ossification the laying down of bone in soft tissue

Horner's syndrome paralysis of the cervical portion of the sympathetic chain resulting in contracted pupil or ptosis of the eyelid

hydrocolloid an occlusive dressing which combines with moisture to form a gel-like substance allowing for moist wound healing

hydronephrosis dilatation of the kidney

hyperreflexic spastic, hypertonic

hypesthesia diminished sensation

incomplete injury partial preservation of sensory and/or motor function below neurological level including lowest sacral segment

incontinence inability to control bowel or bladder elimination

induration hard, swollen area below skin surface

intermittent mandatory ventilation (IMV) spontaneous ventilation intermittently augmented by positive pressure ventilation at mandatory intervals

intermittent positive pressure breathing (IPPB) therapeutic application of inspiratory positive pressure to airway via mask or mouthpiece

intravenous pyelogram (IVP) a radiographic profile of the kidneys

ipsilateral same side

irrigate to cleanse a body area by flushing with fluid

laminectomy a surgical procedure done to remove vertebral arch to gain access to and view the spinal cord

lithotripsy (extracorporeal shock wave lithotripsy) a non-surgical technique to crush and evacuate kidney and bladder calculi

lower motor neuron (LMN) lesion injury below L_1, characterized by a flaccid paralysis

magnetic resonance imaging (MRI) a diagnostic tool used to demonstrate cord compression and hemorrhage

micturition voiding, urinating

myelogram radiographic study performed to determine patency of spinal canal

myelotomy division of connections between anterior and posterior horns

myositis ossificans excess calcium deposits in muscle tissue

nephron structural and functional unit of the kidney

neurectomy interruption of the peripheral nerve

neurogenic having origin in the nervous tissue

neuron basic functional and anatomical unit of central nervous system

orthosis external supportive device

osteomyelitis infection of bone

osteoporosis weakness of bone

paraparesis weakness of lower extremities

paraplegia paralysis of lower extremities

periarticular ossification (PAO) deposits of calcium around joint

phlebography radiographic examination that provides visualization of veins after injection of contract material

plexus intricate network of nerves

pneumobelt an inflatable abdominal corset for assisted ventilation

poikilothermia disruption of thermoregulation caused by autonomic nervous system, cardiovascular system and hypothalamic changes

positive and expiratory pressure (PEEP) a setting on mechanical ventilators that maintains pressure above atmospheric at end of expiration; helps to prevent alveolar collapse

priapism persistent abnormal erection of penis

profilometer an instrument used to measure bladder capacity and response to stimuli

proprioception positional awareness

pulmonary function tests (PFTs) series of tests used to evaluate ventilatory diffusion and perfusion abilities

quadriparesis weakness of all four extremities

quadriplegia paralysis of all four extremities

reflex arc path that an impulse travels from receptor to effector organ; reflex is resulting action

reflux condition where urine backs up through ureters

renal ultrasound a noninvasive procedure using sound waves to assess kidney function

rhizotomy division of anterior and posterior spinal nerves

SEP's (somatosensory evoked potential) a measurement of sensory impulses; used to determine the extent of injury and prognosis

spasm involuntary muscle contraction

sphincter a small muscle that can open or occlude a passageway, for instance in the urethra or anus

sphincterotomy surgical resection of external urethral sphincter to facilitate urine flow from bladder

spinal shock areflexic state resulting from sudden cessation of efferent impulses

stereognosis the ability to recognize an object by touch

stress a condition where the person's emotional or physical equilibrium is threatened

tenodesis movement in the wrist that results in the natural opposition of thumb and forefinger

tenodesis split hand orthosis that uses the natural wrist extension to provide pinch grasp

TENS (transcutaneous electrical nerve stimulation) electrical stimulation of nerve fibers blocking the transmission of pain

tomogram radiographic study that provides segmental visualization of target area

T-piece special tracheostomy adapter to provide humidified air or oxygen

transfer method of moving from one surface to another

transurethral resection (TUR) surgical procedure that removes some of bladder neck tissue to facilitate urine flow

upper motor neuron (UMN) lesion injury above L_1, resulting in a hypertonic paralysis

ureter tube connecting each kidney to the bladder

urethra communicating passageway between bladder and perineum

vasomotor shock (neurogenic) state of massive vasodilatation with hypotension and bradycardia secondary to loss of sympathetic tone

APPENDIX I

RESOURCE PHONE NUMBERS

The following organizations (telephone numbers included) provide information on SCI related concerns.

Accent On Information, (309) 378-2961

American Coalition of Citizens with Disability, (202) 628-3470

American Paralysis Association, (800) 225-0292, (201) 379-2690

Association for Advancement of Rehabilitation Technology, (202) 857-1199

AT&T Office on Devices for People with Disabilities, (800) 233-1222

AT&T Special Needs Center, (800) 833-3232

Center on Education and Training, (800) 848-4815

Center for Health Promotion and Education Hotline, (404) 329-3492

Center for Rehabilitation Technology Hotline, (404) 894-4960

Clearing House for the Handicapped, (202) 730-1245

Disability Rights Center, (202) 223-3304

ERIC Clearinghouse on Adult Career and Vocational Education, (800) 848-4815

HEATH (Higher Education and Adult Training for People with Handicaps), (800) 544-3248, (202) 939-9320

Independent Living Research Utilization, (713) 797-0200

Information Center for Individuals with Disabilities, (617) 727-5540

Inspector General's Hotline Department of Health and Human Services, (800) 368-5779, (301) 597-0724

Institute for Rehabilitation Disability Management, (202) 547-6644

Medicare Medicaid Complaint Line, (800) 368-5779, (301) 597-0724

Miami Project to Cure Paralysis, (800) 782-6387

National Association of Medical Equipment Suppliers, (703) 836-6263

National Association of the Physically Handicapped, (614) 852-1664

National Association of Rehabilitation Facilities, (703) 556-8848, (301) 654-5882

National Handicapped Sports and Recreation Association, (301) 652-7505

National Health Information Clearinghouse, (800) 336-4797, (703) 522-5290

National Health Information Center Hotline, (800) 336-4797

National Information Center for Children and Youth with Disabilities, (800) 999-5599

National Injury Information Clearinghouse Hotline, (301) 492-6424

National Institutes of Health, (301) 496-5751

National Library Services for the Blind and Physically Handicapped, (202) 287-5100

National Organization on Disability, (202) 293-5960

National Paraplegic Foundation, (312) 346-4779

National Rehabilitation Association, (703) 836-0850

National Rehabilitation Information Center, (800) 346-2742

National Spinal Cord Injury Association, (800) 962-9629

National Spinal Cord Injury Hotline, (800) 526-3456

National Wheelchair Athletic Association, (303) 632-0698

Paralyzed Veterans of America, (800) 232-1782, (202) 872-1300

President's Committee on Employment of the Handicapped Hotline (202) 653-5044

Rehabilitation Services Administration Department of Education, (202) 732-1282

Research and Training Center on Independent Living, (913) 842-7694

Society for the Advancement of Travel for the Handicapped, (718) 858-5483

Spinal Network, (800) 338-5412

Stifel Paralysis Research Foundation, (800) 225-0292

Society for the Advancement of Travel for the Handicapped, (718) 858-5483

Spinal Network, (800) 338-5412

Stifel Paralysis Research Foundation, (800) 225-0292

United Organization of Persons with Disabilities, (602) 882-5476

Vocational Instructional Materials Laboratory, (800) 848-4815

World Institute on Disability, (415) 486-8314

APPENDIX II

SPINAL CORD INJURY CENTERS

Georgia Regional SCI System
Shepherd Spinal Center
2010 Peachtree Road, NW
Atlanta, GA 30309
(404) 352-2020

Midwest Regional SCI System
Northwestern University Medical Center
250 East Chicago Avenue,
Suite 619
Chicago, IL 60611

Mount Sinai SCI Model System
One Gustave L. Levy Place
New York, NY 10029
(212) 241-9657

Northern California SCI System
Santa Clara Valley Medical
Center
751 South Bascom Avenue
San Jose, CA 95128
(408) 299-5643

Northern New Jersey SCI
System
Kessler Institute for
Rehabilitation
1199 Pleasant Valley Way
West Orange, NJ 07052
(201) 731-3600, ext. 250

Northwest Regional SCI
System
Rehabilitation Medicine,
University of Washington
1959 N.E. Pacific Street
Seattle, WA 98195
(206) 543-8171

Regional SCI System of Delaware Valley
Thomas Jefferson Hospital
111 South 11th Street
Philadelphia, PA 19107
(215) 955-6573

Regional SCI Care System of
Southern California
Rancho Los Amigos Medical
Center
7601 East Imperial Highway
Downey, CA 90242
(310) 940-7167

Rocky Mountain Regional SCI
System
Craig Hospital
3425 South Clarkson Street
Englewood, CO 80110
(303) 789-8220

Southeast Michigan Regional
SCI System
Wayne State University
261 Mack Boulevard
Detroit, MI 48201
(313) 745-9731

Texas Regional SCI System
The Institute for Rehabilitation
and Research
Texas Medical Center
1333 Moursund Avenue
Houston, TX 77030
(713) 797-5910

University of Alabama, Birmingham SCI Care System
1717 6th Avenue South
Birmingham, AL 35233
(205) 934-3330

University of Michigan Model
SCI System
University of Michigan
Hospitals
300 North Ingalls Building
Ann Arbor, MI 48109
(313) 763-0971

Augusta VAMC
2460 Wrightsboro
August, GA 30910
(404) 724-5116

Brockton VAMC
940 Belmont Street
Brockton, MA 02401
(617) 583-4500

Bronx VAMC
130 Kingsbridge Road
Bronx, NY 10468
(212) 584-9000

Castle Point VAMC
Castle Point, NY 12511
(914) 831-2000

Cleveland VAMC
10701 East Boulevard
Cleveland, OH 44106
(216) 791-3800

East Orange VAMC
Tremont Avenue
East Orange, NJ 07019
(201) 676-1000

Hampton VAMC
2115-1A Executive Drive
Hampton, VA 23667
(804) 722-9961

Hines VAMC
Fifth and Roosevelt Road
Hines, IL 60141
(708) 343-3878

Houston VAMC
2002 Holcombe Boulevard
Houston, TX 77030
(713) 795-4411

Jefferson Barracks VAMC
St. Louis, MO 63129
(314) 487-0400

Long Beach VAMC
5901 East Seventh Street
Long Beach, CA 90822
(213) 494-2611

Memphis VAMC
1030 Jefferson Avenue
Memphis, TN 48104
(901) 523-8990

Miami VAMC
1201 Northwest 16th Street
Miami, FL 33125
(305) 324-4455

Milwaukee VAMC
5000 West National Avenue
Milwaukee, WI 53295
(414) 384-2000

Palo Alto VAMC
3801 Miranda Avenue
Palo Alto, CA 94304
(415) 493-5000

Richmond VAMC
1201 Broad Rock Boulevard
Richmond, VA 23249
(804) 230-0001

San Juan VAMC
One Veteran's Plaza
San Juan, PR 00927
(809) 758-7575

Seattle VAMC
1660 South Columbian Way
Seattle, WA 98108
(206) 762-1010

Sepulveda VAMC
16111 Plummer Street
Sepulveda, CA 91343
(818) 891-7711

Tampa VAMC
13000 Bruce B. Downs Blvd.
Tampa, FL 33612
(813) 972-2000

West Roxbury VAMC
1400 VFW Parkway
West Roxbury, MA 02132
(617) 323-7700

APPENDIX III

PATIENT FAMILY TEACHING OVERVIEW*

The following generic outline provides an overview of recommended patient and family education topics to be presented in a multi disciplinary format. The details of the content and the order of presentations can then be individualized for each learner.

1. NEUROLOGICAL MANAGEMENT
    A. Spinal Column and Cord Anatomy and Physiology
        1. Describe the anatomy and function of the spinal column.
        2. Describe the anatomy and function of the spinal cord.
    B. Mechanisms and Effects of Injury
        1. Identify the most common causes of SCI.
        2. Describe the mechanisms of spinal cord damage.
        3. Summarize the potential effects of SCI on body functions.
        4. Define spinal shock.
    C. Levels and Types of Injury
        1. Describe the methods for determining sensory, motor and functional levels (with individualized explanations of test results).
        2. Describe key components of the ASIA Impairment Scale.
        3. Define upper motor neuron and lower motor neuron injuries and discuss the effects on function.
        4. Define spinal shock.
    D. Management Methods

---

*Adapted from *Education Guide for Spinal Cord Injury Nurses: A Manual for Teaching Patients, Families and Caregivers M. Hanak (Ed.). AASCIN, NY, 1990.*

       1. Review methods of post injury management.

       2. Discuss special considerations related to the stabilization/immobilization method applicable to the individual. Review recovery potential and research projects.

   E. SCI Related Conditions: Pain

       1. Discuss types of sensations experienced below the level of injury and possible causes.

       2. Discuss pain management measures.

   F. SCI Related Conditions: Impaired Temperature Regulation

       1. Describe temperature regulation pre- and post-injury.

       2. Identify methods to conserve body heat.

       3. Describe methods to reduce body heat.

   G. SCI Related Conditions: Autonomic Hyperreflexia (Dysreflexia)

       1. Define autonomic hyperreflexia.

       2. Identify who is susceptible.

       3. Describe the course of autonomic hyperreflexia.

       4. Identify conditions that can cause or increase susceptibility to autonomic hyperreflexia.

       5. Describe the common signs and symptoms of autonomic hyperreflexia.

       6. Review management measures.

       7. Identify six steps to help prevent autonomic hyperreflexia.

II. CARDIOVASCULAR MANAGEMENT

   A. Circulatory System Anatomy and Physiology

       1. Describe the basic structures and functions of the circulatory system.

       2. Describe factors that affect and promote normal blood flow from the veins to the heart.

       3. Describe how the circulatory system is affected by SCI.

   B. Potential Problems

       1. Discuss signs, causes, and prevention/treatment of deep vein thrombosis.

       2. Discuss signs, causes, and prevention/treatment of lower extremity edema.

3. Discuss signs, causes, and prevention/treatment of orthostatic hypotension.
  C. Demonstrations/Practice Sessions
      1. Positioning to help prevent DVT and lower extremity edema.
      2. Application of elastic stockings and binder.
III. Respiratory Management
  A. Respiratory System Anatomy and Physiology
      1. Describe the basic structures and functions of the respiratory system.
      2. Describe the process of breathing.
      3. Define three terms used to describe respiratory status.
      4. Discuss how respiratory function is affected by SCI.
  B. Respiratory Treatment and Support Measures
      1. Discuss the signs, causes and prevention/treatment measures of respiratory infections.
      2. Discuss mechanical ventilation management and precautions.
      3. Discuss alternative measures for respiratory support and their precautions.
  C. Demonstration/Practice Sessions
      1. Assisted cough.
      2. Postural drainage positions.
      3. Clapping and percussion.
      4. Tracheostomy care and suctioning.
      5. Ventilator care.
      6. Phrenic pacer care.
      7. Pneumobelt care.
IV. NUTRITION
  A. Dietary Components
      1. Identify the key components of balanced nutrition.
      2. Describe the function of each component.
      3. Identify food sources for the above.
  B. Mechanical Considerations
      1. Describe mechanical problems which may interfere with chewing or swallowing.
      2. Identify methods to alleviate such problems.

C. Physiologic Considerations
   1. Identify four gastrointestinal changes which affect nutrition.
   2. Describe changes in the genitourinary system which require nutrition intervention.
   3. Describe metabolic changes after SCI.
   4. Discuss the implication of nutrition with skin care.
D. Psychological and Cultural Considerations
   1. Discuss the psychological factors which may affect nutrition.
   2. Identify strategies for corrective actions.
   3. Discuss the implications of cultural beliefs on dietary habits.
V.   BLADDER MANAGEMENT
A. Urinary Tract Anatomy and Physiology
   1. Describe the basic structures and functions of the urinary tract.
   2. Describe the process of micturition (urination).
   3. Discuss how bladder function is affected by SCI.
   4. Describe the goals of a successful bladder management program.
B. Factors That Promote Successful Bladder Management
   1. Discuss the role of effective and regular bladder emptying in successful bladder management.
   2. Discuss fluid intake in relation to bladder management.
   3. Discuss diet and its role in bladder management.
   4. Discuss the importance of physical activity in successful bladder management.
   5. Discuss the importance of adequate personal hygiene and urinary appliance care.
   6. Identify and discuss the purposes, precautions and/or side effects of prescribed bladder medications.
C. Potential Problems
   1. Discuss signs, causes and prevention/treatment of urinary tract infections.

    2. Discuss signs, causes, and prevention/treatment of detrusor sphincter dyssynergia.

    3. Discuss signs, causes and prevention/treatment of autonomic hyperreflexia.

    4. Discuss signs, causes and prevention/treatment of urinary calculi.

    5. Discuss signs, causes and prevention/treatment of hydronephrosis.

    6. Discuss signs, causes and prevention/treatment of reflux.

VI.   **BOWEL MANAGEMENT**

  A. Digestive Tract Anatomy and Physiology

    1. Describe the basic structures and functions of the digestive tract.

    2. Describe the process of defecation.

    3. Discuss how bowel function is affected by SCI.

    4. Describe the goals of a successful bowel management program.

  B. Factors that Promote Successful Bowel Management

    1. Discuss the role of regularity and timing in successful bowel management.

    2. Discuss diet and its role in bowel management.

    3. Discuss fluid intake in relation to bowel management.

    4. Discuss prescribed bowel medications and when and how to make changes in medications and schedules.

    5. Discuss the importance of positioning and physical activity in successful bowel management.

  C. Potential Problems

    1. Discuss signs, causes and prevention/treatment of constipation.

    2. Discuss signs, causes and prevention/treatment of impaction.

    3. Discuss signs, causes and prevention/treatment of diarrhea.

    4. Discuss signs, causes and prevention/treatment of hemorrhoids.

  D. Demonstrations/Practice Sessions

    1. Suppository insertion.

        2. Digital stimulation.

        3. Manual evacuation.

VII.   SKIN CARE

    A.   Skin Anatomy and Physiology

        1. Describe the structure and function of the skin.

        2. Describe the effects of SCI on the skin.

        3. Identify factors contributing to skin breakdown.

    B.   Factors that Promote Skin Health

        1. Describe how to maintain healthy skin through adequate diet and fluid intake and review individual dietary and fluid intake patterns.

        2. Discuss pressure relief measures to use in the wheelchair and bed.

        3. Discuss the purpose and elements of skin inspection.

        4. Describe how to increase skin tolerance.

        5. Describe how to maintain healthy skin through appropriate hygiene measures.

        6. Discuss the importance of wearing proper clothing.

        7. Discuss ways to prevent frostbite and burns.

        8. Discuss the effects of psychological factors on skin maintenance program.

    C.   Demonstrations/Practice Sessions

        1. Skin inspection.

        2. Wheelchair weight shifts.

        3. Bed and wheelchair positioning.

VIII.   MUSCULOSKELETAL CONSIDERATIONS

    A.   Spasticity

        1. Define spasticity.

        2. List precipitating factors for spasticity.

        3. List the benefits of spasticity.

        4. List the potential problems related to spasticity.

        5. Describe methods for reducing and/or managing spasticity.

        6. List additional management methods for treating severe spasticity. Review in depth any methods applicable to the individual patient.

    B.   Skeletal System Changes

        1. Discuss signs, causes and prevention/treatment of osteoporosis and pathological fractures.

        2. Discuss signs, causes and prevention/treatment of heterotopic ossification.

   C.   Technological Advances

        1. Discuss technological advances appropriate to various types of paraplegics.

        2. Discuss technological advances appropriate to various types of quadriplegics.

   D.   Demonstrations/Practice Sessions

        1. Range of motion and stretching exercises.

        2. Application of orthoses.

        3. Technological devices.

        4. Activities of daily living.

IX.   PSYCHOLOGICAL ADJUSTMENT TO SPINAL CORD INJURY

   A.   Managing Stress

        1. Define stress and identify the signs, symptoms and causes.

        2. Discuss the relationship between stress and disability.

        3. Review questions to assist in self evaluation of coping strengths and weaknesses.

        4. Discuss stress management techniques and coping strategies.

   B.   Communication

        1. Discuss the variables that can interfere with effective communication.

        2. Describe an assertive person.

        3. Review factors involved in assessing communication and behavior style.

        4. Discuss methods to enhance listening skills.

        5. Provide guidelines for enhancing communication skills.

   C.   Self-Image

        1. Discuss the components that create a person's self-image.

        2. Discuss the factors that may impact on a person's self-image following SCI.

        3. Review questions to assist in self-assessment.

    4. Provide guidelines to help in achieving supportive self dialogue.

    5. Provide guidelines for improving interpersonal skills.

  D. Demonstrations/Practice Sessions

    1. Relaxation exercises.

    2. Communication techniques.

    3. Social skills training.

X. SEXUAL CONSIDERATIONS

  A. Sexuality

    1. Define sexuality.

    2. Discuss multiple components including body image, beliefs, goals, attitudes and relationships with others.

    3. Discuss patient and partner concerns related to # 2, and enhancement and clarifying strategies.

  B. Sexual Anatomy and Physiology

    1. Identify the structures of sexual function and their purposes.

    2. Discuss the male and female sexual response cycles.

    3. Discuss the effects of SCI on sexual function.

    4. Discuss the effects of SCI on fertility.

  C. Management of Physical Concerns

    1. Review contraceptive options.

    2. Discuss safe sexual practices.

    3. Discuss compensatory measures for decreased vaginal lubrication in females.

    4. Discuss surgical and non-surgical treatments for erection impairments in males.

    5. Discuss mobility and positioning options.

    6. Discuss sensory enhancements and compensatory measures.

    7. Discuss measures to prevent bowel and bladder interferences.

    8. Discuss effects of medication on sexual response.

    9. Discuss relationship between hyperreflexia and sexual activity.

          10. Discuss methods of sexual enhancement and alternatives.

XI.   DISCHARGE PREPARATION

    A.   Medications and Supplies

        1. Discuss pertinent information regarding prescribed medications.

        2. List the considerations when selecting a medical supply vendor.

        3. List possible sources for obtaining a medical supply vendor.

        4. Discuss what medical supplies will be needed after discharge.

        5. Discuss the necessary steps to obtaining medical supplies after discharge.

    B.   Follow-Up Care

        1. State the purposes of follow-up care.

        2. Identify team members in after care program.

        3. Review information needed for the first follow-up visit.

    C.   Emergency Medical Care

        1. Identify each individual's local hospital/emergency room and the family physician after discharge.

        2. List possible emergency situations and identify potential solutions.

    D.   Community Resources

        1. Discuss access to public education, vocational resources, and employment considerations.

        2. Identify national SCI resources and facilities.

        3. Discuss access to public transportation.

        4. Discuss how to obtain insurance.

        5. Discuss sports and recreation opportunities.

        6. Discuss how to obtain information on accessible travel.

BIBLIOGRAPHY

Abrams, P. (1985). Detrusor instability and bladder outlet obstruction. *Neurology and Urodynamics, 4*:317–328.

Ader, K., Pierce, L., & Salter, J. (1990). Urinary tract infections: Quality assurance rehabilitation nursing perspectives. *Rehabilitation Nursing, 15*(4), 193–196.

Alderman, M. (1978). Setting a chronic pain treatment program: Ridding the pain patient of chemical crutches. *Patient Care, 12*, 74–75, 102–103.

Alfin-Slater, R., & Krutcherski, D. (1980). *Nutrition and the adult: Micronutrients*. New York: Plenum Press.

Allen, M. S. (1984). Nursing care of the spinal cord patient with recurrent pressure sores. *Journal of Rehabilitation Nursing, 9*(1), 34–36.

American Spinal Injury Association. (1989). *Pain in SCI: Epidemiology, neurophysiology and clinical management*. Ann Arbor: University of Michigan Medical Center.

American Spinal Cord Injury Association. (1992). *Standards for neurological and functional classification of spinal cord injury patients*. Chicago: American Spinal Cord Injury Association.

Apple, D., & Hudson, L. (Eds.). (1990). The SCI model: Lessons Learned and new applications. *Proceedings of the National Consensus Conference on Catastrophic Illness and Injury*. (pp. 66–81, 104–105, 109–122). The Georgia Regional SCI Care System, Shepherd Center for Spinal Injuries, Atlanta, GA.

Bell, J., & Hannon, K. (1986). Pathology involved in autonomic dysreflexia. *Journal of Neuroscience Nursing, 18*(2), 86.

Bennett, J., Gray, M., Greene, G., & Foote, J. (1992). Continent diversion and bladder augmentation in spinal cord injured patients. *Seminars in Urology, 10*(2), 121–132.

Berczeller, P., & Bezkor, M. (1986). *Medical complications of quadriplegia*. Chicago: Yearbook Medical Publishers.

Block, R., & Basbaum, M. (Eds.). (1986). *Management of spinal cord injuries*. Baltimore: Williams and Wilkins.

Boroch, R. (1979). *Elements of rehabilitation in nursing*. St. Louis: C. V. Mosby Co.

Bradley, W. (1986). Physiology of micturition. In P. Walsh, R., Gitles, A. Perlmutter, & T. Stamey, *Campbell's Urology*. Philadelphia: W. B. Saunders Company.

Braken, M., et al., (1990). A Randomized controlled trial of methylprednis olone and Naloxone in the treatment of acute spinal cord injury. *New England Journal of Medicine, 322*, 1405–1411.

Braun, R. (1978). *Tender mercies*. New York: Alfred A. Knopf.

Brickner, R. (1976). *My second twenty years, an unexpected life*, New York: Basic Books.

Brown, D., Judd, F., & Unger, G. (1987). Continuing care of the spinal cord injured. *Paraplegia, 25*(3), 296–300.

Brown, M., Gordon, W., & Ragnarsson, K. T. (1987). Unhandicapping the disabled: What is possible? *Archives of Physical Medicine and Rehabilitation, 68*(4), 206–209.

Buchanan, L., & Narvoczenski, D. (Eds.). (1987). *Spinal cord injury: Concepts and management approaches*. Baltimore: Williams and Wilkins.

Burke, D., & Morray, D. (1975) *Handbook of spinal cord medicine*. New York: Raven Press.

Cardenas, D., Kelly, E., Krieger, J., & Chapman, W. (1988). Residual urine volumes in patients with spinal cord injury: Measurement with a portable ultrasound instrument. *Archives of Physical Medicine and Rehabilitation, 69*(7), 514–516.

Carter, E. R. (1987). Respiratory aspects of spinal cord injury. *Paraplegia, 25*, 252–262.

Chantraine, A. (1979–1980). Clinical investigation of bone metabolism in spinal cord lesions. *Paraplegia, 17*, 253.

Chu, D., Ahn, J., Ragnarsson, K. T., Helt, J., Folcarelli, M. A., & Ramirez, A. (1985). Deep vein thrombosis: Diagnosis in spinal cord injured patients. *Archives of Physical Medicine and Rehabilitation, 66*(6), 365–368.

Cioschi, H. (1987). Alterations in urinary elimination. *Application of Rehabilitation Concepts to Nursing Practice*. (2nd ed.) Evanston, IL: Rehabilitation Nursing Foundation.

Claus-Walker, J., Campos, J. R., Carter, R. E., Vabona, C., & Liscomb, H. S. (1972). Calcium excretion in quadriplegia. *Archives of Physical Medicine and Rehabilitation, 53*, 1.

Comarr, A. (1966). Observations on menstruation and pregnancy among female spinal cord injury patients. *Paraplegia, 3*, 263.

Comarr, A., & Vigue, M. (1978). Sexual counseling among male and female patients with spinal cord injury and/or Cauda Equina Injury. *American Journal of Physical Medicine, 57*, 107.

Comfort, A. (1978). *Sexual consequences of disability*. Philadelphia: George F. Stickley.

Cristopherson, V., Coulter, P., & Wolanin, M. (1974). *Rehabilitation nursing: Perspectives and application*. New York: McGraw-Hill.

Cyr, L. (1989). Sequelae of SCI after discharge from the initial rehabilitation program. *Rehabilitation Nursing, 14*(6), 326–329.

Davidoff, G., Morris, J., & Roth, E. (1985). Cognitive dysfunction and mild closed head injury in traumatic spinal cord injury. *Archives of Physical Medicine and Rehabilitation, 66*, 489–491.

DeLisa, J. A., (Ed.). (1988). *Rehabilitation medicine*. Philadelphia: J. B. Lippincott.

deToledo, L. (1980). Caring for the patient instead of the ventilator. *RN, 43*(2), 20.

DeVivo, M. J., & Fine, P. R. (1986). Predicting renal calculus occurrence in SCI patients. *Archives of Physical Medicine and Rehabilitation, 67*(10), 722–725.

Demitrijevic, M. M. (1986). Spinal cord stimulation for the control of spasticity in patients with chronic spinal cord injury: Clinical observations. *Central Nervous System Trauma, 3*(2), 129–144.

Eisenberg, M., Griggins, C., & Duval, R. (1982). *Disabled people as second-class citizens*. New York: Springer.

Eisenberg, M., & Rustad, L. (1976). Sex education and counseling program on a spinal cord injury service. *Archives of Physical Medicine and Rehabilitation, 57*, 135.

El Ghatit, A. (1975). Outcome of marriages existing at the time of spinal cord injury in males. *Chronic Disease, 7*, 383.

El Ghatit, A., & Hansen, R. (1976). Marriage and divorce after spinal cord injury. *Archives of Physical Medicine and Rehabilitation, 57*, 470.

Fife, D., & Krause, J. (1986). Anatomic location of spinal cord injury— relationship to the cause of injury. *Spine, 11*(1), 2–5.

Folotico, J. (1987). Pulmonary embolism. *RN, 42*(2), 47–51.

Ford, R. D., & Duckworth, B. (1987). *Physical management of the quadriplegic patient* (2nd ed.). Philadelphia: V. A. Davis.

Frye, B. (1986). A model of wellness-seeking behaviors in traumatic spinal cord injury victims. *Rehabilitation Nursing, 11*(5), 6–7.

Fuchs, P. (1979). Understanding continuous mechanical ventilation. *Nursing, 79, 9*(12), 26–33.

Gabrielson, M. A. (May 14, 1985). How injuries occur and what approaches might be appropriate to reduce injuries. *National Pool and Spa Safety Association Conference*.

Ganong, W. F. (1989). *Review of medical physiology*, (14th ed.). Norwalk, CT: Appleton and Lange.

Gaumer, W. (1979). Electrical stimulation in chronic pain. *American Journal of Nursing, 3*, 504.

Gilman, A. G., Rall, T. W., Nies, A. S., & Taylor, P., (Eds.). (1990). *Goodman and Gilman's the pharmacological basis of therapeutics* (8th ed.). New York: Pergamon Press.

Goldfinger, G., & Hanak, M. (Eds.). (1979). *Spinal cord injury: A Guide for care.* New York: New York Spinal Cord Injury Center.

Gray, M. (1992). *Genitourinary disorders.* Clinical Practice Series. St. Louis: C. V. Mosby.

Griffith, E., & Trieschmann, R. (1975). Sexual functioning in women with spinal cord injury. *Archives of Physical Medicine and Rehabilitation, 56*, 18.

Guha, A., Tator, C. H., Endrenyl, L., & Piper, I. (1987). Decompression of the spinal cord improves recovery after acute experimental spinal cord compression injury. *Paraplegia, 25*, 324–339.

Guttman, L. (1976). *Spinal cord injury system, Comprehensive management and research.* (2nd ed.). Oxford, England: Blackwell Scientific Publications.

Guyton, A. C. (1991). *Textbook of medical physiology* (8th ed.). Philadelphia: W. B. Saunders Company.

Hackler, R., Hall, M., & Zampieri, T. (1989). Bladder hypecompliance in the SCI population. *Journal of Urology, 141*(6), 1390–1393.

Hamilton, S. (1987). Sexuality and disability. In *Application of rehabilitation concepts to nursing practice* (pp. 189–192). Evanston: Rehabilitation Nursing Foundation.

Hammond, M. C., Umlauf, R. L., Matteson, B., & Perduta-Fulginiti, F. (Eds.). (1989). *Yes, you can! A guide to self-care for persons with spinal cord injury.* Washington, DC: Paralyzed Veterans of America.

Hanak, M. (1986). Patient and family education. New York: Springer.

Hanak, M. (1992). *Rehabilitation nursing for the neurological patient.* New York: Springer.

Hancock, D., et al. (1979–1980). Bone and soft tissue changes in paraplegic patients. *Paraplegia, 17*, 267.

Hart, J. (1981). Spinal cord injury: Impact on clients' significant others. *Rehabilitation Nursing, 11-18.* January–February.

Ireland, F. (1976). *Spinal cord injury care manual for nurses.* New York: Eastern Paralyzed Veterans Association.

Johnson, R., et al. (1977). Cervical orthoses. *Journal of Bone and Joint Surgery, 59A*, 332–339.

Katz, R. T. (1988). Management of spasticity. *American Journal of Physical Medicine and Rehabilitation, 67*(3), 108–116.

Kerr, A. (1980). *Orthopedic nursing procedures: Part I* (3rd ed.). New York: Springer.

Killen, J. (1990). Role stabilization in families after spinal cord injury. *Rehabilitation Nursing, 15*(1), 19–21.

Kirshblum, S., & Zafonte, R. (September 6–8, 1989). Dangers of elastic bandage immobilization of the spinal cord injury patient. *Abstracts Digest*, Annual Meeting, American Spinal Cord Injury Association. Las Vegas.

Kleinfield, S. (1979). *The Hidden Minority, America's Handicap*. Boston: Little, Brown.

Kohke, F. J., & Lehman, J. F., (eds.). (1990). *Krusen's handbook of physical medicine and rehabilitation* (4th ed.). Philadelphia: W. B. Saunders.

Kunkel, C. F., Scremin, E., Eisenberg, B., Garcia, J. F., Roberts, S., & Martinez, S. (1993). Effect of standing on spasticity, contracture and osteoporosis in paralyzed males. *Archives of Physical Medicine and Rehabilitation, 74*(1), 73–78.

Lamid, S. (1988). Long-term follow-up of spinal cord injury patients with vesicourteral reflux. *Paraplegia, 26*(1), 27–34.

Lamphier, T. (1981). Upper gastrointestinal hemorrhage: Emergency evaluation and management. *American Journal of Nursing, 9*, 1814–1817.

Lappe, F. (1975). *Diet for a small planet*. New York: Ballantine Books.

Laven, G., Huang, C., DeVivo, M., Stover, S., Kuhlemeier, K., & Fine, P. (1989). Nutritional status during the acute stage of spinal cord injury. *Archives of Physical Medicine and Rehabilitation, 70*(Apr), 277–282.

Lazare, J. N., Saltzman, B., & Sotolongo, J. (1988). Extracorporeal shock wave lithotripsy treatment of spinal cord injury patients. *Journal of Urology, 140*(2), 266–269.

Lazure, L. (1980). Defusing the dangers of autonomic dysreflexia. *Nursing 80, 10*, 52–54.

Lee, M., Mathews, P., & Yarkony, G. (1989). Rehabilitation of quadriplegic patients with phrenic nerve pacers. *Archives of Physical Medicine and Rehabilitation, 70* (July), 549–552.

Lindan, R., Leffler, E., & Freehafer, A. (1990) The team approach to urinary bladder management in SCI patients. A 26-year retrospective study. *Paraplegia, 28*(5), 314–317.

Lloyd, E., Toth, L., & Perkash, I. (1989). Vacuum tumescence: An option for spinal cord injured males with erectile dysfunction. *SCI Nursing, 6*(2), 25–28.

Lloyd, L. K. (1986). New trends in urologic management of SCI patients. *Central Nervous System Trauma, 3*(1), 3–13.

Lloyd, L., Kuhlemeier, K., Fine, P., & Stover, S. (1986). Initial bladder management in spinal cord injury: Does it make a difference? *Journal of Urology, 135*(Mar), 523–527.

Martin, N., Holt, N., & Hicks, D. (Eds.) (1981). *Comprehensive rehabilitation nursing.* New York: McGraw-Hill.

Maynard, F., & Muth, A. (1987). The choice to end life as a ventilator-dependent quadriplegic. *Archives of Physical Medicine and Rehabilitation, 68*(Dec), 862–864.

McCagg, C. (1988). Postoperative management and acute rehabilitation of patients with spinal cord injuries. *Orthopedic Clinics of North America, 17*(1), 171–182.

McGuire, F., & Savastano, J. (1986). Comparative urological outcomes in women with SCI. *Journal of Urology, 135*(4), 730–731.

Mechner, F. (1976). Patient assessment: Neurological examination, Part III. *American Journal of Nursing, 76*, 1–25.

Midwestern Regional Spinal Cord Injury Center, Acute Spinal Cord Injury Trauma Unit. (1977). *Spinal cord injury: A Handbook for physicians, nurses and other medical professionals.* Chicago, IL: MRSCIC.

Miller, H. J., Thomas, E., & Wilmot, C. (1988). Pneumobelt use among high quadriplegic population. *Archives of Physical Medicine and Rehabilitation, 69*, 369–372.

Morris, J., Roth, E., & Davidoff, G. (1986). Mild closed head injury and cognitive deficits in spinal cord injured patients: Incidence and impact. *Journal of Head Trauma Rehabilitation, 1*, 31–42.

Moses, R., et al. (1979). Does the MA–1 respirator make you nervous? *RN, 41*(2),   .

Mount Sinai Hospital. (1992). *Policies and procedures for pressure sores*, New York City, NY.

Naftchi, E., et al. (1980). Mineral metabolism in spinal cord injury. *Archives of Physical Medicine and Rehabilitation, 61*, 39.

Naftchi, E., et al. (1980). Spinal cord injury: Effect of thyrocalcitonin on calcium, magnesium and phosphorus in paraplegic cats. *Archives of Physical Medicine and Rehabilitation, 61*, 515.

National Research Council. (1980). *Recommended dietary allowances.* Washington, D.C.: National Academy of Sciences.

Nelson, A. (1990). Patients' perspectives of a spinal cord injury unit. *SCI Nursing, 7*(3), 44–63.

Nelson, A. (1987). Normalization: The key to integrating the spinal cord injured patient into the community. *SCI Nursing, 4*(1), 3.

Nickel, V., & Pierce, D. (1977). *The total care of spinal cord injuries.* Boston: Little, Brown.

Nielson, C. (1980). Mechanical ventilation. *American Journal of Nursing, 80*, 2191.

Norton, L. C., & Neureuter, A. (1988). Weaning the long-term ventilator dependent patient: Common problems and management. *Critical Care Nurse, 9*(1), 42–52.

Oakes, D. (1990). Benefits of an early admission to a comprehensive trauma center for patients with SCI. *Archives of Physical Medicine and Rehabilitation, 72*(9) 637–643.

Ozer, M. (1988). The management of persons with SCI. New York: Demos Publication.

Ozer, M., & Shannon, S. (1991). Renal sonography in asymptomatic persons with SCI: A cost effective analysis. *Archives of Physical Medicine Rehabilitation, 72*(1), 35–37.

Parke, B., & Penn, R. D. (1989). Functional outcome after delivery of intrathecal baclofen. *Archives of Physical Medicine and Rehabilitation, 70*, 30–32.

Penn, R. D., & Kroin, J. S. (1987). Long-term intrathecal baclofen infusion for treatment of spasticity. *Journal of Neurosurgery, 66*, 181–185.

Pettin, A., & Carolan, J. (1981). How to stop a GI bleed. *RN, 4*, 43.

Phillips, L., Ozer, M., Axelson, P., & Chizeck, H. (1987). *Spinal cord injury: A guide for patients and family*. New York: Raven Press.

Phipps, W. J., Long, B. C., Woods, N. F., & Cassemeyer, V. L. (Eds.). *Medical–surgical nursing: Concepts and clinical practice*. St. Louis: Mosby Year Book.

Pires, M. (1989). Substance abuse: The silent saboteur in rehabilitation. *Nursing Clinics of North America, 24*(1), 291–296.

Purin-Parkinson, C. (1979). Sorting out adrenergic-cholinergic drugs. *RN, 7*, 52–54.

Rabin, B. (1980). *The sensuous wheeler: Sexual adjustment for the spinal cord injured*. San Francisco: Multimedia Resource Center.

Rehabilitation Nursing Foundation. (1987). *Rehabilitation nursing concepts and practice—A core curriculum* (2nd ed.). Skokie, IL: Author.

Richards, J., Brown, L., Hagglund, K., Bua, G., & Reeder, K. (1988). Spinal Cord injury and concomitant traumatic brain injury: Results of a longitudinal investigation. *American Journal of Physical Medicine and Rehabilitation, 67*(5), 211–226.

Rucker, B., Szasz, G., & Carpenter, C. (1988). Legal, ethical and religious issues related to fertility enhancements of men with spinal cord injuries. *Canadian Journal of Rehabilitation, 1*(4), 225–231.

Rutecki, B., & Seligson, D. (1980). Caring for the patient in a halo apparatus. *Nursing 80, 9*, 73.

Santosh, L., Hamilton, B. B., Heinemann, A., & Betts, H. B. (1986). Risk factors for heterotopic ossification in spinal cord injury. *Archives of Physical Medicine and Rehabilitation, 70*(May), 387–390.

Stover, S., & Fine, P. (1986). *Spinal cord injury: The facts and figures.* Birmingham, AL: National Spinal Cord Injury Research Data Center, University of Alabama.

Stryker, R. (1979). *Rehabilitation aspects of acute and chronic nursing care.* Philadelphia: W. B. Saunders.

Suddath, D. S. (1991). *Lippincott manual of nursing practice* (5th ed.). New York: J. B. Lippincott Co.

Task Force in Concerns of Physically Disabled Women. (1978). *Within reach: Toward intimacy.* New York: Human Sciences Press.

Trieschmann, R. (1988). *Spinal cord injuries, psychological, social and vocational adjustment.* New York: Demos Publications.

Trieschmann, R. (1987). *Aging with a disability.* New York: Demos Publications.

Tucker, S. (1980). The psychology of spinal cord injury: Patient–staff interaction. *Rehabilitation Literature, 41,* 714.

Tyson, G., et al. (1978). *Acute care of the head and spinal cord injury patient in the emergency department.* Charlottesville, Virginia: Department of Neurosurgery, University of Virginia.

U.S. Department of Health & Human Services. (May, 1992). *Clinical practice guideline, pressure ulcers in adults: Prediction and prevention.* Rockville, MD: Author.

U.S. Department of Health & Human Services. (March, 1992). *Clinical practice guideline, urinary incontinence in adults.* Rockville, MD: Author.

Vash, C. (1981). *The psychology of disability.* New York: Springer.

Wanner, M. B., Rageth, M. D., & Zach, G. A. (1987). Pregnancy and autonomic hyperreflexia in patients with spinal cord lesions. *Paraplegia, 25,* 482–490.

Whiteneck, G., et al. (1989). *The management of high quadriplegia.* New York: Demos Publications.

Williams, J. M., & Kay, T. (Eds.). (1990). *Head injury, a family matter.* Baltimore: Paul H. Brooks Publishing Co.

Williams, L. (1989). Pharmacologic erection programs: Treatment option for erectile dysfunction. *Rehabilitation Nursing, 14*(5), 264–268.

Wilmot, C. B., Cope, D. N., Hall, K. M., & Acker, M. (1985). Occult head injury: Its incidence in spinal cord injury. *Archives of Physical Medicine and Rehabilitation, 66,* 227–231.

Winterhalen, J. G. (1992). Group support for families during the acute phase of rehabilitation. *Holistic Nursing Practice, 6*(2), 23–31.

Wright, B. (1960). *Physical disability: a psychosocial approach.* New York: Harper.

Wyndaele, J. (1987). Urethral sphincter dyssynergia in spinal cord injury. *Paraplegia, 25*(1), 10–15.

Young, R. R., & Delwaide, P. J. (1981). Drug therapy, spasticity. Parts I and II. *New England Journal of Medicine, 304*(1), 28, *304*(2), 96.

Zejdlik, C. P. (1992). *Management of spinal cord injury* (2nd ed.). Boston: Jones & Bartlett Publications.

INDEX

SP *Springer Publishing Company*

REHABILITATION NURSING FOR THE NEUROLOGICAL PATIENT

Marcia Hanak, BSN, MA, CCRN

Here is a practical new reference written especially for practicing nurses who work with neurologically disabled persons. Hanak emphasizes the interrelation of rehabilitation and wellness in this thorough, medical approach to rehabilitation nursing.

Contents:

I. Overview • Wellness Promotion • Patient and Family Education • Neuroanatomy and Physiology Review

II. Nursing Management of Problems Common to Neurorehabilitation • Neurogenic Bladder Management • Neurogenic Bowel Management • Dysphagia Management • Sexuality and Disability

III. Nursing Management of Specific Neurological Disabilities • Traumatic Brain Injury Management • Spinal Cord Injury Management • Cerebral Vascular Accident Management • Multiple Sclerosis Management • Amyotrophic Lateral Sclerosis Management • Parkinson's Disease Management • **Appendixes** • Psychosocial Discharge Planning References • Resource Phone Numbers

240pp   0-8261-7660-7   hardcover

536 Broadway, New York, NY 10012-3955 • (212) 431-4370 • Fax (212) 941-7842

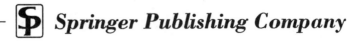

Springer Publishing Company

PATIENT AND FAMILY EDUCATION
Teaching Programs for Managing Chronic Disease and Disability

Marcia Hanak, BSN, MA, CRRN

What makes up an effective patient education program? This volume provides an easily accessible guide focusing on the nurse's role. Chapters span chronic disease/health care management, disability management, psychosocial considerations, and evaluation/documentation tools. Specific coverage includes common childhood illnesses, diabetes mellitus, arthritis, cerebral palsy, Guillan-Barré syndrome, spina bifida, stress management for patients, and a patient education profile.

"...well written, carefully researched, extremely accurate ... a valuable resource." —Rehabilitation Nursing

Partial Contents:

I. OVERVIEW: Introduction • Patient and Family Education Guidelines

II. CHRONIC DISEASE AND HEALTH CARE MANAGEMENT: Cardiovascular Diseases • Common Childhood Illnesses and Emergency Management • Chronic Obstructive Pulmonary Disease • Diabetes Mellitus • Seizure Management

III. DISABILITY MANAGEMENT: Arthritis • Cerebral Palsy • Cerebral Vascular Accident • Head Trauma • Lower Extremity Amputation • Multiple Sclerosis • Parkinson's Disease Spinal Cord Injury

IV. PSYCHOSOCIAL CONSIDERATIONS: Stress Management Teaching Guide • Sexual Considerations

V. EVALUATION AND DOCUMENTATION TOOLS: Learning Assessment Guides • Teaching Checklist

Translated into Spanish

272pp   0-8261-5441-7   softcover

536 Broadway, New York, NY 10012-3955 • (212) 431-4370 • Fax (212) 941-7842

Springer Publishing Company

HEALTH ASSESSMENT OF THE OLDER INDIVIDUAL, 2nd Ed.

Mathy D. Mezey, EdD, FAAN
Louise M. Rauckhorst, MSN, RN   NEW EDITION
Shirlee A. Stokes, EdD, RN

"An excellent guide for nurses caring for older adults in any setting. It covers a broad spectrum, including theories of aging, developmental changes, and sociocultural changes as well as health and illness assessment skills....This book belongs in every clinical nurse's personal library."
—**Geriatric Nursing**

Contents:

The Role of Assessment in the Care of the Older Person

Growth and Development of the Older Person

Interviewing for the Health History

Functional Assessment

Assessment of General Appearance, Skin, Hair, Feet, Nails, and Endocrine Status

Assessment of Changes in the Eye, Ear, Nose, Mouth, and Neck

Assessment of the Cardiac, Vascular, Respiratory, and Hematopoietic Systems

Assessment of Nutritional Status, Gastrointestinal Functioning, and Abdominal Examination

Assessment of Sexual, Genital, and Urinary Functioning

Musculoskeletal Assessment

Assessment of Mental/Emotional Status

Assessment of Neurological Functioning

Assessment of Community, Home, and Nursing Home

Changes in Laboratory Values and Their Implications

Appendix: Key Health Status Objectives Targeting Older Adults

256pp   0-8261-2902-1   hardcover

536 Broadway, New York, NY 10012-3955 • (212) 431-4370 • Fax (212) 941-7842

Springer Publishing Company

KEY ASPECTS OF COMFORT
Management of Pain, Fatigue, and Nausea

Sandra G. Funk, PhD,
Elizabeth M. Tornquist, MA,
Mary T. Champagne, PhD, RN,
Laurel A. Copp, PhD, RN, FAAN, and
Ruth A. Wiese, MSN, RN, Editors

The maintenance of patient comfort is at the very core of nursing care. This extraordinary book distills the most up-to-date and groundbreaking research on patient comfort into a readable jargon free format.

Partial Contents:

I. Key Aspects of Comfort.

II. Pain In Infants and Children. Acute Pain Behavior in Infants and Toddlers • The Oucher: A Pain Intensity Scale for Children • The Accuracy of Nurses' and Doctors' Perceptions of Patient Pain • The Effect of Music on Adult Postoperative Patients' Pain During a Nursing Procedure.

III. Fatigue. Fatigue in Patients with Catastrophic Illness • Fatigue in Women Receiving Chemotherapy for Ovarian Cancer.

IV. Nausea. Nausea and Vomiting in Pregnancy • The Effectiveness of Self-Care Actions in Reducing "Morning Sickness".

V. Comfort. Perceptions of Comfort by the Chronically Ill Hospitalized Elderly • Fatigue, Pain, Depression, and Sleep Disturbance in Rheumatoid Arthritis Patients

Nurses' Book Society Main Dual Selection

352pp   0-8261-6760-8   *hardcover*

536 Broadway, New York, NY 10012-3955 • (212) 431-4370 • Fax (212) 941-7842

Springer Publishing Company

KEY ASPECTS OF ELDER CARE
Managing Falls, Incontinence, and Cognitive Impairment

Sandra G. Funk, PhD,
Elizabeth M. Tornquist, MA,
Mary T. Champagne, PhD, RN,
and **Ruth A. Wiese,** MSN, RN, Editors

This volume looks at three particular areas of concern for the elderly—falls, incontinence, and cognitive impairment. These are key problems for the elderly in acute and long-term care settings and at home. Any of them threatens the elderly's independence and quality of life; together they represent major obstacles to continued functioning.

368pp   0-8261-7720-4   hardcover

536 Broadway, New York, NY 10012-3955 • (212) 431-4370 • Fax (212) 941-7842